MW00768360

Fundamentals of
Research Methodology
for Health Care Professionals

Fundamentals of
Research Methodology
for Health Care Professionals

Second edition

Hilla Brink

revised by

Christa van der Walt

Gisela van Rensburg

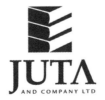

JUTA
AND COMPANY LTD

Fundamentals of Research Methodology
for Health Care Professionals

First published 1996
Second edition 2006
Reprinted 2007

© Juta & Co. (Pty) Ltd
PO Box 24309
Lansdowne
Cape Town
7779

This book is copyright under the Berne Convention. In terms of the Copyright Act, No. 98 of 1978, no part of this book may be reproduced or transmitted in any form or by any means, electronic or mechanical, including photocopying, recording or by any information storage and retrieval system, without permission in writing from the Publisher.

ISBN 0 7021 6680 4
ISBN 978 0 7021 6680 8

Editing and proofreading by Danya Ristić
Cover design by Alexander Kononov
Index by Cecily van Gend
DTP and design by Charlene Bate
Printed and bound by Mills Litho, Maitland, Cape Town, South Africa

Contents

CHAPTER 3

Ethical considerations in the conduct of health sciences research

CHAPTER 4

An overview of the research process

CHAPTER 5
Selecting or identifying research problems

CHAPTER 6
The literature review

CHAPTER 7

Refining and defining the research question or formulating a hypothesis and preparing a research proposal

CHAPTER 8

Quantitative research

CHAPTER 11

Data collection

CHAPTER 12

Data quality

Chapter 13
Data analysis

Chapter 14
Research reports and report evaluation

Preface

Fundamentals of Research Methodology for Health Care Professionals is intended specifically for health care professionals and undergraduate students who are taking an introductory course in research. Its major purpose is to provide information about the logic of scientific enquiry generally, to guide novice researchers through the research process, and to stimulate awareness of the myriad researchable and research-needed questions encountered in daily practice.

This text is not intended as a comprehensive, in-depth source which provides all the answers relating to the research process; it should be seen, rather, as a stepping stone to more sophisticated textbooks. It emphasises using and applying research, and provides conceptual and non-technical descriptions of the methods used by researchers. It not only covers the steps of the research process, but also explains what a researcher does and provides a guide to evaluating each of the steps in the research process. The steps are illustrated with examples from practice. Both qualitative and quantitative approaches are integrated in the text. The most common methods used in quantitative and qualitative research are presented and illustrated with examples from practice.

Each chapter contains chapter outcomes, examples, summaries, and exercises specific to the chapter content to facilitate understanding and assimilation of the information provided. An extensive glossary includes both qualitative and quantitative research terminology to assist the reader in evaluating research reports and in becoming acquainted with the terminology used in the text.

We believe that this new edition will continue to be an invaluable source to novice researchers.

Hilla Brink
Christa van der Walt
Gisela van Rensburg

1 Orientation to health sciences research

LEARNING OUTCOMES

On completion of this chapter, you should be able to demonstrate your understanding of

- research, and health sciences research
- ways of acquiring knowledge
- the scientific method of enquiry
- the main types of health sciences research
- the differences between the major features of qualitative and quantitative research
- the differences between and the similarities of the research process and the problem-solving process
- reasons for conducting health sciences research
- the various roles of health care professionals in research
- evidence-based practice.

Introduction

Research is important for any profession. In fact, it is frequently referred to as the 'lifeblood', the 'hallmark' or the 'cornerstone' of the development of a profession. Every professional needs knowledge on which to base his/her practice, and scientific knowledge provides a particularly solid foundation. As Ottenbacher (1990) states, "in a true profession, the skills come from a clearly defined and well-developed knowledge base, generated largely by members of the discipline". Christiansen (1981) warns that the failure of health care professionals to meet the challenge of research may ultimately lead to the demise as viable disciplines. True also of the health sciences, this fear has been expressed by many health care scholars and organisations.

We must accept research as an integral part of health care practice, education and management, and that 'research-mindedness' should be fostered in health care professionals from the beginning of their training. Professionals must be aware of and knowledgeable about the application of research in their practice.

This book intends to orientate you to the field of health sciences research, to equip you with basic research skills, and to assist you in becoming an enthusiastic researcher and a critical consumer of research findings.

What is research?

The term 'research' is used in various ways by so many people that we often accept it without considering exactly what it means. In the vernacular, research has come to signify almost any sort of information gathering or checking. As valuable as it may be, such activity is not research as defined by the scientist. In science, research refers to exploration, discovery and careful study of unexplained phenomena. It is suggested that we can distinguish the vernacular and scientific definitions by emphasising the first syllable of the word when we mean the former process (*re*search), and the second syllable of the word when we mean the latter process (re*search*) (Ahrens 1992, Burns & Grove 2005).

For the purpose of this book the term 'research in the health sciences' is used to signify the latter definition. In the literature, you will find a wide variety of definitions of scientific research. Table 1.1, opposite page, provides three of these. With regard to the above definitions, we can identify the following characteristics of research:

- The result of research is an *increase in knowledge*, which in turn contributes to the existing body of knowledge. The ultimate aim of research in the health care sciences is to provide strong evidence on which the practice of quality care can be based (Burns & Grove 2005).
- There is at least one method by means of which this knowledge is obtained, be it *search, discovery or enquiry*. This implies that the researcher is actively involved in

Table 1.1 Definitions of research		
Some definitions of research		
The systematic investigation into and study of materials, sources, etc., in order to establish facts and reach new conclusions. An endeavour to discover new or to collate old facts by the study of a subject or by a course of critical investigation (Reader's Digest Oxford Complete Wordfinder 1993: 1306)	An attempt to increase the sum of what is known, usually referred to as a body of knowledge, by the discovery of new facts or relationships through a process of systematic scientific enquiry, the research process (Macleod-Clark & Hockey 1989: 4)	Diligent systematic enquiry to validate and refine existing knowledge and generate new knowledge (Burns & Grove 2005: 2)

looking for information which as yet is not readily available or for which there is no generally accepted evidence.

- The search is *systematic and diligent*, which implies planning, organisation and persistence. The researcher proceeds in an orderly manner, according to a logical, predetermined scheme, and tries to minimise the likelihood that results will be influenced by faults in the apparatus or in the methodology, or by his/her expectations (Burns & Grove 2005; McConway 1994).
- Research is a *process*, which implies that there should be a purpose, a series of actions and a goal. The purpose gives direction to the process, and the series of actions are organised into steps to achieve the identified goal.
- Research is a *scientific process*; in other words, it is the systematic way of applying the scientific method. Science as a process implies orderly, logical and public activity. 'Public' in this context means that research findings, and the methods used to acquire them, are made known to members of the research community. It is therefore important that the researcher reports every step in the research process in detail, so as to enable other researchers to evaluate and repeat the enquiry in another context. Furthermore, the scientific process implies precision, accuracy and lack of bias. It also involves scepticism, which means that unconfirmed observations, propositions or statements – even when made by great authorities – are open to refutation and analysis, and need to be confirmed. The researcher must provide evidence or logical justification in support of his/her conclusions or statements of fact, so that they can be scrutinised by other researchers. Though it is impossible for the researcher to exert total control, the scientific method nevertheless implies that he/she should attempt to exercise as much control as possible over the research situation – to increase the reliability and validity of the research findings.

What is health sciences research?

Research in the health sciences is multidimensional in that it is concerned with clinical research, education, management, ethics, historical research, legislation and social aspects related to health care sciences. Thus it spans a wide field of investigation.

This is consistent with the definition of nursing research which was approved by the International Council of Nurses (ICN) in 1987. According to the ICN,

> nursing research focuses on developing knowledge of the care of persons in health and illness. ... It also emphasises the generation of knowledge of policies and systems that effectively and efficiently deliver nursing care; the profession and its historical development; ethical guidelines for the delivery of nursing services and systems that effectively and efficiently prepare nurses to fulfil the profession's current and future social mandate.

Although not much has been written on research in the other health professions, it is clear that the divergent opinions among researchers regarding the definition of research do not affect the definition of research itself. In terms of the research process, the same rules of the scientific method apply and the same series of logical steps, which the researcher must undertake to develop the current knowledge base, are used by *all* disciplines, including the health care sciences. The disagreement in the health care profession is about what constitutes a legitimate subject for investigation; in other words, of what the area of concern for health care researchers should comprise.

Ways of acquiring knowledge

The scientific method of enquiry is not only an essential element of research, it is also generally considered to be the most sophisticated and reliable way of acquiring knowledge. However, it is only *one* source of health care knowledge. Through the years, health care professionals have come to rely on several sources of knowledge to guide their practice. Before we begin to explore the scientific method in detail, we now briefly discuss alternative sources of knowledge, which as a means of contrast may be useful in illuminating the specific characteristics of the research process.

Tradition

Knowledge can be handed down from one generation to the next. It leads to action that occurs because 'it has always been done that way'. There are certain advantages. Each researcher need not begin anew in the attempt to understand the world or an aspect of the world. Tradition also facilitates communication, because it provides a common frame of reference for each member of an investigative group. However, tradition also poses some problems. Many traditions have never been evaluated for validity. They may also contribute to stagnation of practice instead of encouraging innovation. This leads to a ritualisation of practice, in which the basis becomes inflexible and developments in the field are rejected without examination.

An example drawn from midwifery illustrates the difference between practice based on common traditional knowledge and that based on research evidence. When it was discovered that specific micro-organisms caused infection under certain conditions, it was assumed that harmful micro-organisms existed in pubic hair. The practice of perineal and pubic shaving before childbirth was introduced to reduce the risk of infection. The practice continued unchallenged for many years, even though it used valuable staff time and resources, and caused some discomfort. However, during the 1970s research showed that there is no increase in infection if the pubic hair is *not* removed (Bond 1980; Romney 1980). Thus, the reduction of infection is no longer an adequate justification for shaving the hair. The professionals who continue the practice today do so in support of the traditional practice, while those who have stopped the practice evidently are aware of and subscribe to these findings.

Authority

Much of health care practice is guided by knowledge obtained from authorities. Authorities are persons with specialised expertise, experience or power in the field who are able to influence opinion and behaviour. Supervisors, instructors and, of course, statutory health care bodies establish policies and procedures that dictate the ways in which health care professionals are to practise. Students turn to teachers or textbooks for answers. The textbook authors are either experts themselves, or they consult experts in order to ensure that their texts contain the correct and necessary information. Such reliance on authorities is to some extent inevitable, because we cannot all become experts on every problem with which we are confronted.

However, while few students and subordinates question the word of the authorities, as a source of information authorities have certain limitations. For instance, the statements of one authority may be contradicted or refuted by another, equally prestigious authority. How can we resolve the conflicting claims? In practice, unless we can find objective and acceptable criteria for resolution, there will be ongoing disputes, slanderous commentary or even aggressive behaviour.

Logical reasoning

We can develop a solution to many a perplexing problem by means of logical reasoning. We can think through a problem using a process of either induction or deduction, or both. Both systems are useful as a means of understanding and organising phenomena, and both play a role in the scientific approach. Neither system, however, is without limitations when used *by itself* as a basis of knowledge.

Inductive reasoning is the process of developing generalisations from specific observations. In other words, with this type of reasoning the researcher obtains facts through observation and makes generalisations based upon these facts. For example, a physiotherapist observes that certain patients in a spinal ward seem to be more anxious than the other patients. Through discussions with all the patients, she discovers that the anxious patients have little knowledge of their medical condition and its implications and expected outcomes, whereas the calmer patients are aware of what their condition involves. She thus concludes that ignorance of one's condition contributes to a high degree of anxiety. She uses inductive reasoning to reach that conclusion. She has observed the phenomenon of anxiety in certain patients, she has interviewed them and the others, and she has come to a conclusion based on her findings.

The disadvantage of inductive reasoning is that the knowledge arrived at through this process is highly dependent upon the representativeness of the specific examples used as a basis for the generalisation. The reasoning process itself offers no mechanism for evaluating this criterion and has no built-in checks for the truth of the conclusion.

Deductive reasoning is the process of developing specific observations from general principles. In other words, with this type of reasoning the researcher moves from a general premise (point of departure) to a particular situation or conclusion. For example, if we believe that any person who experiences the loss of a close family member will grieve, then we may conclude that because Caroline Jones's husband has died, she will grieve. We use deductive reasoning to apply a general principle to a specific case.

Deductive reasoning can also lead to an erroneous conclusion, since the validity of the reasoning is dependent upon the truth of the general premise on which the prediction is based. Cultural stereotypes, for example, can be the basis of faulty reasoning. If a health care professional bases a therapeutic approach to the case of a Greek patient on the erroneous premise that all Mediterranean people are hot-headed and emotional, serious misjudgements may result. Clearly, the limitation of deductive reasoning is that it works practically only if we have means for establishing the veracity of the general principle.

Nevertheless, both deductive and inductive reasoning are important in the development of knowledge. As Streubert Speziale and Carpenter (2003) point out, the researcher will select an inductive or a deductive stance or a combination of both, depending on the research question.

Experience

Our experience represents a familiar and functional source of knowledge. Although it is often said that 'there is no teacher like experience', this approach has its drawbacks. An individual's experience may be too restricted to allow for generalisations about new situations to be developed. Furthermore, each person tends to experience or perceive an event differently. A person's experiences are coloured by his/her values and prejudices.

Trial and error

Closely related to experience is the method of trial and error. Trial and error is similar to informal experimentation. A researcher encounters a problem, attempts an intervention and, if the intervention works, he/she adopts it as a solution. If it does not work, the researcher tries alternate approaches until he/she finds a suitable solution.

While this method may offer a practical means of securing knowledge, it is often fallible and inefficient. It also tends to be haphazard, and it may not be possible for other researchers to repeat the experiment.

Intuition

We sometimes acquire knowledge in a sudden insight, which arises without our conscious reasoning. For instance, you wake up in the middle of the night with a creative answer to a problem that you spent days trying to solve. Intuitive 'leaps' in science and the arts, made by Einstein and Beethoven, for example, have lead to significant contributions to humanity. Unfortunately, at times even the most impressive intuition is proven false when put to an empirical test. Therefore, intuition is generally considered to be an insufficient means of approaching information in a research context. We should not forget, however, that it can serve as a guiding and creative addition.

Borrowing

According to Burns and Grove (2005), borrowing in health sciences involves the appropriation and use of knowledge from other fields or disciplines. Over the years, the health care sciences have borrowed in two ways. First, some health care professionals have taken information from disciplines such as medicine, sociology, psychology, physiology and education, to name but a few, and applied it directly to their practice. But this information was not integrated into the unique focus of health care sciences. Second, borrowing has entailed the integration of information from other disciplines into the focus of health care sciences.

As with the other methods, borrowing can be problematic, particularly if the researcher does not understand the context from which he/she borrows ideas, theories or evidence. When information is used out of context, significant distortion may result. Borrowed knowledge, therefore, is not necessarily adequate for answering questions generated in health care practice.

The scientific method

Having examined certain ways of obtaining knowledge, we can contrast these with the scientific method. Table 1.2 summarises the differences between the features of the scientific method and other methods of acquiring knowledge.

Table 1.2 Key features of the scientific method and other methods	
The scientific method	**Alternative methods**
Uses empirical enquiry (data are collected by means of observation via the human senses)	May accept fanciful explanations
Uses a systematic approach (i.e. the researcher moves in an orderly fashion through a series of steps according to a predetermined plan of action)	May use haphazard and unsystematic approaches
Makes empirical data public (i.e. all steps and findings are recorded precisely and in an unbiased manner and published or presented to fellow researchers so that they can be checked and verified)	Are frequently not recorded or documented or shared in other ways
Uses control and objectivity (i.e. the investigator uses checks and mechanisms to minimise the possibility of biases and confounding factors)	Make little or no attempt to control variables
Strives for the development of conceptual explanations or theories	Select evidence from personal experiences or performances
Strives for generalisability	Often focus on isolated events
Tends not to deal with metaphysical explanations that cannot be empirically tested	May be highly metaphysical or spiritual
Uses tested reasoning (verification and falsification) or justification	Are frequently based on rituals

Controversies and limitations of the scientific method

Despite the commonly accepted principles of the scientific method of enquiry, scientists differ in their view of science itself. Some scientists have rigid views, while others are more open and relativistic in their outlook. This has caused much debate, controversy and change. For example, traditionally it was held that science presents us with proven knowledge and the absolute truth. But there is sufficient evidence today that tells us that this is not so. Instead, what we refer to as 'knowledge' is provisional and based on the best available current understanding in the field.

Science is changing all the time, just as it continually challenges our commonly held beliefs and ideas, and proposes new ones. Thus it is imperative that, before embarking on a new research project, a researcher ascertains the currently held views of his/her chosen topic, as well as the accepted methods of investigation.

Traditionally, natural science also assumes that the scientist and the object of study are separate, and that the object is governed by laws and rules that do not vary. The scientist's behaviour and values, moreover, do not influence the discovery of knowledge. Scientific knowledge is thus taken as value-free. More recently, by contrast, scientists have begun to acknowledge that their findings may be influenced by their own ideas and viewpoints, which cannot (and should not) be ignored or eliminated for the convenience of research. Although they strive to be objective and to minimise the influence of personal factors, scientists now recognise that these factors may never be eradicated entirely. In the past, researchers adhered strictly to the rigid rules of natural science. Today, health scientists feel that the traditional view is incompatible with the philosophical views of humanism and holism to which they subscribe.

Phenomenologists have argued that the traditional scientific approach, rooted as it is in logical positivism, is overly reductionistic and cannot adequately capture the human experience in all its complexities. Other limitations of the approach are that it inadequately provides answers to moral or value-laden questions, and that much of human behaviour is too complex to be measured by the conventional instruments of science (Polit, Beck & Hungler 2001). Consequently, ideas about what is legitimate for the health care sciences have broadened, and a shift from the fixed view of science to a more liberal one is now occurring.

Main types of scientific research

Research is categorised according to point of view and purpose. The most basic distinction found in textbooks is between applied and basic, or pure, research. Burns and Grove (2005) point out that this distinction is made according to the major aim of the researcher. When the researcher seeks to develop theories that increase knowledge, he/she will engage in **basic** or **pure research**, while when he/she aims to solve problems or make decisions for what are considered practical purposes, he/she will conduct **applied research.**

Research is designed to achieve the maximum degree of control and thus to support the validity of the study. In light of this, the researcher should ask him-/herself: 'Is there an intervention or not?' This leads to the classification of research into two broad categories, namely, experimental and non-experimental research.

Within experimental designs you will find two sub-types, namely, the true experiment and the quasi-experiment. The **true experimental approach** has three characteristics:

1 Manipulation of the independent variable.
2 Control over the experimental situation by the researcher.

3 Randomisation, which means giving every subject an equal chance of selection when assigning subjects to a control group or an experimental group after the subjects have been randomly selected from the target population.

The **quasi-experimental approach** is similar to the true experimental approach except that it lacks either all the characteristics of randomisation or control over the experimental situation.

The **non-experimental approach** covers other kinds of research, in which manipulation of the independent variable is impossible, not to mention inappropriate, and/or the other experimental approaches are impractical or inappropriate. One of the most practical classifications of non-experimental research is based on the *purpose* of research. Burns and Grove (2005) suggest the following classification:

■ **Descriptive designs.** This includes typical descriptive designs, comparative descriptive designs and case studies. These designs can further be described according to the time sequence in which the data are collected, as follows:

❑ **Retrospective** (or *ex post facto*) designs measure variables that have occurred in the past.

❑ **Prospective** designs measure variables that will occur during the course of the study.

❑ The time frame that the researcher uses also dictates whether the design is **longitudinal**, which describes a design that follows subjects over time, or **cross-sectional**, which describes a study that the researcher conducts in the present to examine that which currently exists.

■ **Correlational designs.** These aim to examine relationships among variables. There are three types of correlational designs: descriptive, predictive and model-testing designs.

Many textbooks distinguish between two broad research approaches: **quantitative** and **qualitative**. The former is said to have its roots in logical positivism and to focus on measurable aspects of human behaviour, while the latter seems to have its roots in symbolic interactionism, or phenomenology, and concentrates on qualitative aspects such as meaning, experience and understanding (Burns & Grove 2005; Polit, Beck & Hungler 2001).

According to Streubert Speziale and Carpenter (2003), qualitative research is characterised by six principles:

1 Believing in multiple realities.
2 Being committed to identifying an approach to understanding that supports the phenomenon studied.
3 Being committed to the participants' viewpoints.
4 Conducting the enquiry in a way that limits disruption of the natural context of the phenomenon of interest.

5 Acknowledging the participants in the research process.
6 Reporting the data in a literary style rich with participant commentaries.

Table 1.3 presents a summary of the major distinguishing features of quantitative and qualitative research.

Table 1.3 Distinguishing features of quantitative and qualitative research	
Quantitative	**Qualitative**
Focuses on a relatively small number of concepts (concise and narrow)	Attempts to understand the phenomenon in its entirety, rather than focusing on specific concepts (complex and broad)
Begins with preconceived ideas about how the concepts are interrelated	Has few preconceived ideas and stresses the importance of people's interpretations of events and circumstances, rather than the researcher's interpretation
Uses structured procedures and formal instruments to collect information	Collects information without formal structured instruments
Collects information under conditions of control	Does not attempt to control the context of the research, but rather attempts to capture that context in its entirety
Emphasises objectivity in the collection and analysis of information	Assumes that subjectivity is essential for the understanding of human experience
Analyses numeric information through statistical procedures	Analyses narrative information in an organised, but intuitive, fashion
Investigator does not participate in the events under investigation – is most likely to collect data from a real distance	Involves sustained interaction with the people being studied in their own language, and on their own turf
Incorporates logistic, deductive reasoning	Inductive and dialectic reasoning are predominant

Source: Based on Burns and Grove (2005), Polit, Beck and Hungler (2001)

The types of research studies we have discussed here present an overview of the major types generally described in current textbooks; you should not see these types as all-inclusive. Furthermore, note that the categories are not mutually exclusive – in practice the differentiation between the types is often less than clear-cut. Various combinations of these categories are possible, as well as the addition of more groups or variables to the basic design. You can regard the categories we have discussed as tools to guide the choice of a research design. The appropriate type that the researcher will select depends on the research problem and the knowledge about it that currently exists.

Many health care professionals and researchers believe that research and problem-solving are synonymous, or even extensions of each other. This is not so. Although there are similarities between the two, there are also key differences. Both problem-solving and research involve identifying a problem area, establishing a plan, collecting data and evaluating the data. A systematic approach and the logical progression of ideas are therefore common to both. The purposes of the two, however, are quite different. **Problem-solving** seeks a solution to an immediate, actual problem that exists for a person or people in a given setting. Application of the results of problem-solving is limited to the setting in which it is conducted and to the individuals within that setting. The purpose of **scientific research** is much broader: the research seeks to obtain knowledge that can be generalised to other people and other settings, or is simply applicable *across* groups. Furthermore, the research problem must be positioned in the context of what has already been discovered – this is called the 'literature review' – and be grounded in a theoretical framework.

Reasons for conducting health sciences research

We cannot over-stress the importance of research in the health sciences. Health care professionals can no longer base their practice on tradition, rituals and unquestioned principles; rather, they must be motivated to become intelligent users of research and research team members. To develop motivation, they need to consider the place of research in professional practice and be convinced that research provides sound information on which they can base changes for the improvement of patient care.

Reasons for health care professionals to conduct research are as follows:

- Improving health care.
- Earning and defending a professional status.
- Establishing scientifically defensible reasons for health care activities.
- Providing other health care professionals with an increasing repertoire of scientifically defensible intervention options.
- Finding ways of enhancing the cost-effectiveness of health care activities.
- Providing a basis for standard-setting and quality assurance.
- Providing evidence of weaknesses and strengths in health care.
- Providing evidence in support of demands for resources in health care services.
- Providing a basis for self-correction of misinterpretations and myths (Hockey 1991; Nieswiadomy 1993).

These reasons are worthy of urgent pursuit, and underscore the fact that research in health sciences is *every* health care professional's business.

Roles of health care professionals in research

Every health care professional should make it a priority to participate in research. This does not necessarily mean *conducting* research – he/she can participate in a variety of other ways.

He/she can

■ act as a member of a research team, assisting in identifying problem areas in health care services or in the collection of data within an established, structured format
■ undertake an independent research project
■ identify and evaluate research findings applicable to the field
■ be a user of research findings
■ act as a patient advocate, when a patient is involved.

While it is possible for novice researchers to conduct small-scale survey-type studies, education beyond the baccalaureate level is necessary for independent researcher status.

Every health care professional should be involved in the *evaluation* of research findings. As research consumers, these professionals are obliged to familiarise themselves with research findings and determine their usefulness in practice.

Using research knowledge to promote evidence-based practice

In the last 50 years, there has been tremendous development in clinical research. At the same time, the findings of research have been disseminated on a broader basis, such as in journals and electronic databases, on television and at conferences. Burns and Grove (2005) urge that greater emphasis be placed on the use of research findings in practice, with the ultimate aim of the health care sciences becoming evidence-based professions.

Thus, health care professionals are under pressure to improve the evidence-base of their practice. Leaders in the field worldwide accept the value of research and evidence-based practice (EBP), but are concerned about the limited extent to which health care professionals utilise and draw upon research findings to determine or guide their decisions about patient care. In the past, health care consumers seldom questioned health care practices or expressed concern that management protocols were not based on evidence. Whether this acceptance had its source in trust or fear is debatable. However, consumers have become more assertive, and have added to the demand that clinical practice be based on scientific evidence.

The classic story of Semmelweis demonstrates the way in which reflective, questioning and accurately observant practitioners can uncover evidence in their own daily practice which, when acted upon, can improve the quality of health care (Craig & Smyth 2002).

EBP aims to deliver appropriate care in an efficient manner to every patient. It has been described as "*doing the right things right*" (Muir Gray 1997: 18; emphasis added). We adopt the definition of EBP from Sackett, Strauss, Richardson, Rosenberg and Haynes (2000: 1; emphasis added), who state that evidence-based medicine (EBM) "*is the integration of best research evidence with clinical expertise and patient values*". Although this definition initially implicated doctors alone, it is now well recognised that *all* health care professionals have a moral and ethical obligation to ensure that the care they render is based on the best available evidence and is of the highest quality possible.

Best research evidence is gathered from clinically relevant research based on the basic health sciences, as well as from patient-centred clinical research. Although this continues to be a point of debate, the current trend is that qualitative research has a place in this definition.

Clinical expertise means the ability of a health care professional to use his/her clinical skills and experience to identify a patient's unique health problems and needs, his/her values and expectations, and the benefit of potential interventions.

Patient values are the unique preferences, concerns and expectations of each patient. These must be integrated into the clinical decision to serve the patient as well as possible.

EBP consists of these five steps:

1 The health care professional constructs a specific question concerning the care of his/her patient, or group of patients. The question could relate to the diagnosis of the problem, the prognosis or likely outcome, the most effective treatments and the possible side-effects; or it could concern the best method of delivering services to meet the patient's needs.
2 The professional seeks the best evidence to answer the clinical question.
3 He/she evaluates the evidence for its veracity and usefulness in the particular situation on the basis of the quality of the research findings, his/her expertise and experience, and the patient's preferences.
4 He/she implements the plan.
5 He/she evaluates the outcome of the intervention (Reynolds 2001).

In order to practise evidence-based care, a health care professional must develop key skills so that he/she can access and use evidence appropriately. Where evidence is not available, he/she needs to make carefully considered decisions. In the meantime, to ensure that his/her clinical decisions are informed as far as possible by current research evidence, he/she can follow the five-step approach as summarised here:

1 Convert information needs into clear questions.
2 Seek evidence to answer those questions.
3 Evaluate or critically appraise the evidence for its veracity and usefulness.
4 Integrate findings with clinical expertise, patient needs and patient preferences. If appropriate, apply the findings.
5 Evaluate performance, and the outcome of the decision/practice (Sackett et al. 2000: 3–4).

It is essential that research is put into practice. Health care professionals should understand both research and the means of accessing published research, as well as its relevance to their own practice and the service provided to the community. Today, we are faced with informed health consumers who demand efficient and effective care. As health care researchers we must ensure that professionals can properly understand and use the evidence that we make available. Research into practice is much more than merely conducting research projects in practice – it is about doing the right research and ensuring that the findings are valued and implemented (Clifford & Clark 2004).

In the UK, the National Health Service (NHS) Executive Report (1996) proposes three main functions in the achievement of clinical efficacy in practice, namely, inform, change and monitor. It is important to *inform* all health care professionals of the importance of clinical efficacy, and to ensure that they have access to the best available evidence in their field of practice. They also need to be empowered to use this information to review their practice and to make *changes* where necessary. Finally, they must *monitor* and assess the effects of change to ensure that the changes result in improvement of the quality of care (Clifford & Clark 2004).

Although health care professionals in South Africa have been involved in research for many years, the findings were not always disseminated. Publications were rare and the impact on clinical change was insignificant. The last decade has witnessed massive change, leading us to question a profession based on ritual and tradition. There are also several factors, however, that have restricted health sciences research:

- Many health care professionals believe that they know the best way to carry out care. If a particular method has not been problematic, they continue to use it without question.
- Some health care professionals have alienated themselves from the research being carried out in their units.
- A research-based culture continues to be uncommon in the health care professions.
- The quantitative vs. qualitative debate has hindered research.
- Health care professionals are often being used only as data collectors.

We predict that EBP will become more universally accepted in the near future, not only in clinical practice, but also in other fields such as health sciences education and management. More health care professionals will be educated in research methodology, managers will encourage their employees to develop themselves through research, and professionals will work inter-professionally on the basis of shared research understanding. We urge you to read more about the various models for research utilisation that have been developed in research textbooks, such as Burns and Grove (2005). Health care professionals need to accept responsibility and accountability for decision-making processes in planning health care. This requires an understanding based on evidence and research (Renfrew & Proctor 2001).

Summary

This chapter is an introduction to health sciences research. The introduction focused on the importance of research for the health care professions. We paid attention to the meaning of research and health sciences research, and to the concept of science. We discussed the difference between the scientific methods and other methods of obtaining knowledge, after which we described the controversies and limitations of the scientific method.

We then addressed the main types of research from various points of view, distinguishing between the major features of quantitative and qualitative research. We also compared the research process with that of problem-solving. Following our presentation of the reasons for conducting research, we referred to the roles of health care professionals in research and concluded the chapter with a brief exploration of evidence-based practice.

Exercises

Complete these exercises:
1 This chapter outlines the divergent opinions of health care researchers about the accurate definition of health sciences research. Take a position in the controversy and argue your point.
2 Consider one or two facts that you know and trace these back to their source. Is the basis of your knowledge tradition, authority, logical reasoning, experience or scientific research? Justify your answer.
3 Discuss the development of EBP in your profession and identify barriers to the implementation of research in clinical practice.
4 As a researcher you wish to study the health perceptions of women in squatter camps. Indicate whether you think the topic would best lend itself to a qualitative or a quantitative research study. Provide a rationale.

2 Research and theory

LEARNING OUTCOMES

On completion of this chapter, you should be able to demonstrate your understanding of

- theory, paradigm, metaparadigm, philosophy, model, framework, concept, construct and proposition
- four types of theory
- the differences between theoretical and conceptual frameworks
- the steps used in developing a theory
- the steps used in testing a theory
- the relationship between research and theory.

Introduction

In the previous chapter we introduced you to scientific research. We compared the scientific method with other ways of obtaining knowledge, and gave an overview of various aspects of research. In this chapter we focus on *scientific theory*. Research and theory are partners in the same way that research and practice are partners. They are interdependent and inseparable. Research is guided by theory and depends on theory to increase its meaningfulness and generality. Theory is usually not and should never be formulated in a vacuum; rather, it depends on carefully conducted research to give its concepts and propositions scientific credibility.

The nature of scientific theory

Theorising is not an exclusively scientific activity. Theories are ideas that we develop from our observations and that we use every day. For example, if you heat a teapot before putting in the tea, you may make a better tasting cup of tea, or if you establish a rapport with a person, he/she may be more compliant. Our everyday theories, however, do not meet the requirements of science. They are usually not derived systematically, they tend to be haphazard and fallible, and there is always the risk of bias. Often, they cannot be supported by reliable evidence. When testing everyday theories, we tend to ignore data that do not conform to our preconceived ideas.

As used by the scientist, theory includes ideas that are formulated and tested systematically and rigorously, and that can be supported by reliable evidence. The development of scientific theory is a deliberate and conscious activity that scientists undertake according to certain established principles. These theories are judged by the academic community on the basis of strict criteria. As we pointed out in the previous chapter, science is continually challenging commonly held beliefs and opinions, and adding new ones. Theories reflect current understanding, hence they may be changed by new knowledge. Therefore, theories are tentative and must be regularly verified. When a more usable theory is developed, an older, less explanatory theory must be reconsidered and perhaps even abandoned.

By way of an example we refer to two theories of ageing. The **disengagement theory** asserts that people deliberately withdraw, or disengage, from business and social interactions as they grow older. **Activity theory** challenges this notion, proposing instead that older people want to remain active in all parts of their lives and that any withdrawal is against their will – in fact, it is an outcome of discrimination towards the elderly. More recent research on healthy older adults provides support for the activity theory. The theory of disengagement is therefore being partially abandoned in favour of the theory of activity.

Definitions of theory

There are many definitions of the term 'theory' in the health sciences literature. Some are narrow and specific; others are broad and generic. Moreover, several concepts are used interchangeably with the term, such as *conceptual framework, conceptual model, paradigm, metaparadigm, theoretical framework* and *theoretical perspective*. Consequently, when you read about theories, it is important for you to note the terminology used in the texts and to determine precisely how the author used these terms contextually. When using the term or its alternatives yourself, remember to clearly define the context in which you do so.

A common definition of theory is formulated by Chinn and Kramer (1991). According to these writers, theory is a "*systematic abstraction of reality that serves some purpose*" (Chinn & Kramer 1991: 2; emphasis added). They describe each part of the definition as follows: 'systematic' implies a specific organisational pattern, 'abstraction' means that it is a representation of reality, and 'purposes' include description, explanation and prediction of phenomena, as well as control of some reality (Chinn & Kramer 1991: 2). A theory summarises and organises current understanding of a particular phenomenon, and may be systematically tested in the 'real world' by research. Examples of theories with which you may already be familiar are Maslow's theory of human needs, Rosenstock's health belief model, Selye's theory of physiological adaptation to stress, the gate control theory of pain and Pender's health promotion model.

Types of theory

Several varieties of theory are described in the literature, such as *metatheory, grand theory, factor-isolating theory, descriptive theory, practice theory*, and so on. This may add to your confusion about what a theory is, or how abstract it needs to be to be called a theory, unless you know the criteria that are used for categorising theories.

Theories are primarily classified according to purpose or to scope, breadth or level of abstraction. Several writers use the latter classification, and depict the scope or level of abstraction according to hierarchical levels from broad to limited, as illustrated in Figure 2.1 on the next page (Chinn & Kramer 1991; Fawcett 1983; Moody 1990; Walker & Avant 1983; Wilson 1989; Woods & Catanzaro 1988). The highest level depicted in Figure 2.1 is **metatheory**, which is the term used to designate theorising about theory in a discipline and the process of developing theory. Metatheory does not address the substantive content of health sciences, except to define the types of theory appropriate within these disciplines. Its focus is on broad issues, including analysis of the purpose and type of theory needed, and proposal and critique of sources and methods for theory development.

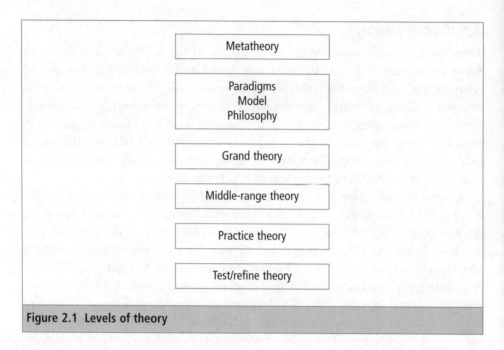

Figure 2.1 Levels of theory

Grand theories provide a global perspective of a discipline and its scope of practice. As a rule, these theories are so abstract that they are not amenable to direct empirical testing. Some writers consider them to be synonymous with conceptual models and paradigms (Moody 1990; Stevens-Barnum 1990). To Merton (1968), a sociologist who first proposed grand and middle-range theories, the former are the core theories of a science and are not testable because they represent conceptual frameworks.

Middle-range theories are less abstract than grand theories and more limited in scope. They usually deal with certain circumscribed phenomena – such as pain, stress, coping mechanisms and chemical dependence – within a clearly defined context. Merton (1968) describes these theories as examining a portion of reality and identifying a few key variables. Propositions are clearly formulated and testable hypotheses can be derived. Middle-range theory is generally more practical, more applicable and more easily tested, confirmed or refuted within the empirical world than is grand theory. Woods and Catanzaro (1988: 22) regard it as the most useful theory for the development of health sciences.

We can distinguish between grand and middle-range theories using an example. Looking at a theory of health or high-level wellness, you would probably note that it represents ideas that have been put together in a unique way to describe or explain health or high-level wellness. Such a theory is evidently useful for the health sciences because it facilitates an understanding of the world in terms of one of the health sciences' major concerns, that is, health. Moreover, it frames the way in which we can view health or high-level wellness and suggests the direction that a research project dealing with related concepts should take. The theory provides a global perspective of health; in other words, it takes into account all of the health care sciences' concern with health and high-level wellness. Therefore, it applies to individuals in general and not to a particular individual in a specific situation. Health and high-level wellness are abstract concepts, and can have various definitions. Thus, the theory that pertains to these concepts is regarded as a grand theory.

By contrast, a theory of pain alleviation or stress management deals with only one part of health sciences' concern with health and high-level wellness. In this theory a definitive piece of reality is suggested in a concrete manner, which is much less obscure than the information provided by a grand theory. The clearer theory is easily tested, confirmed or refuted in the empirical world, and therefore can be called a middle-range theory.

A theory that deals with one person in one situation at one point in time – for example improving regional blood flow, or altering action potential – is described as **narrow-range** or **micro-theory**. Concepts contained in this type of theory are narrow and of limited scope, and are often specifically defined. Such a theory is generally considered to be useless in many health care situations.

Practice theory, the second last type depicted in Figure 2.1, is characterised by its goal of prescriptive action for health care practice. Dickhoff and James (1968: 202) identify four levels of practice theory based on the existing body of knowledge about a phenomenon. The lower levels are developed first, and provide a basis for the higher levels of theory. The levels are as follows:

1   **Factor-isolating theory** focuses on observing, describing and naming concepts. This leads the researcher to construct the factor-isolating or concept-naming theory. This level is also known as the 'descriptive level'.
2   **Factor-relating theory** takes the isolated concepts a step further and relates them to one another. Description is still the purpose of the study, but at this level it focuses on the relationships between the concepts.
3   **Situation-relating theory** explains the interrelationships of the concepts or propositions. The researcher attempts to answer the question, 'What will happen if ...?' and accordingly designs a study to test the relationships.
4   **Situation-producing theory** requires the specification of an activity as well as its goal. This theory is also referred to as a 'prescriptive theory' as it prescribes what the health care professional must do to attain a desired goal. The question here is: 'How can I make this happen?'. Thus the purpose of this level of theory is predictive.

Theory-related terms

As we mention above, there are concepts that are either used interchangeably with the term 'theory' or are closely related to it. The concepts of metaparadigm,

paradigm, models, frameworks and philosophy are growing increasingly popular in the literature that deals with research and theory. As a prospective researcher, you need to become familiar with these terms, which we will now explore. Our focus is on the predominant use of these terms in the literature, though we will indicate cases in which more than one usage is prevalent.

Paradigm

Since the publication of Kuhn's *The Structure of Scientific Revolutions* (1970), the term 'paradigm' has been used with increasing frequency in the scientific community. Kuhn uses the term in many ways. Among others, he defines it as a discipline's specific method of structuring reality (1970). Laudan (1977) describes a paradigm as a set of assumptions about the basic kinds of entities in the world, about how these entities interact, and about the proper methods to use for constructing and testing theories of these entities.

In *The Paradigm Dialogue*, Guba (1990) describes a paradigm as

■ **ontology** – a patterned set of assumptions about reality
■ **epistemology** – knowledge of that reality
■ **methodology** – the particular ways of knowing about that reality.

These assumptions and ways of knowing are untested 'givens' that guide and influence the researcher's investigation. He/she must decide what assumptions are acceptable and appropriate for the topic of interest, and must use methods consistent with that paradigm. Guba (1990) identifies and gives an overview of four paradigms as relevant for researchers, namely, *positivism, post-positivism, critical theory* and *constructivism*. A discussion of these paradigms is beyond the scope of this book; Guba's (1990) text provides adequate description.

According to Moody (1990), a prominent health sciences researcher, a paradigm helps the researcher to be organised in his/her thinking, observing and interpreting processes. In essence, a paradigm frames the way in which a discipline's concerns is viewed, and the direction that a research project takes. For example, it structures the questions that need to be posed, it eliminates questions that are external to the conceptual boundaries of the paradigm, it provides a link to certain types of research methods, and it suggests criteria with which the researcher can judge appropriate research tools and which can be used to evaluate the quality of the research effort.

In simple terms, a paradigm is an overarching philosophical framework of the way in which scientific knowledge is produced. Yet, while the scientific community widely accepts the term, several writers caution that there are also disadvantages in a discipline's acceptance of a dominant paradigm (Feyerabend 1975; Moody 1990;

Wilson 1989). Feyerabend, a historian-philosopher of science, provides two reasons for his position. First, epistemological prescriptions are not a guarantee of the *best* way to discover a few isolated facts or 'secrets' of nature and, second, rigid scientific education cannot be reconciled with a humanitarian attitude. Moody (1990) and Wilson (1989) are also against an unquestioning adherence to a particular paradigm, as they believe that this may blind us to discoveries and delay scientific progress, and make us prisoners of our own paradigms. Concerned as it is with complex human phenomena and social needs, the very nature of health care practice demands not one but *multiple* paradigms for viewing reality and providing structure for systematic study.

Metaparadigm

The term 'metaparadigm' is frequently used in the literature, and is derived from Kuhn's (1970) original work on paradigms. The metaparadigm constitutes the global perspective of a discipline, and serves as an encapsulating unit or framework within which the more defined models, paradigms or theories develop. The metaparadigm of each discipline specifies its distinctive perspective. There appears to be general agreement among scholars that the concepts of *person, health, environment* and *action,* comprise the health sciences' metaparadigms (Bush 1979; Fawcett 1983; Flaskerud & Holloran 1980; Moody 1990; Newman 1983; Wilson 1989; Yura & Torres 1975).

Philosophy

The term 'philosophy' is used in several senses in the literature. In this book we use it to refer to worldview, or *Weltanschauung*. It denotes our assumptions, values and beliefs about the nature of reality, knowledge, methods for obtaining knowledge, ourselves, our health, the health sciences and the environment.

Model

This term is also used inconsistently in the literature. While it often seems synonymous with the term 'theory', some writers distinguish between the two terms and view a model as a *precursor* of a theory (Mouton 1996).

A model is frequently described as a symbolic depiction of reality. It provides a schematic representation of certain relationships among phenomena, and it uses symbols or diagrams to represent an idea. A model helps us to structure the way we can view a situation, event or group of people. In relation to health sciences research, a model may help us to define and guide specific research tasks, or provide an organised framework.

Frameworks

A framework of a research study helps the researcher to organise the study and provides a context in which he/she examines a problem and gathers and analyses data. In much of the literature a distinction is made between theoretical and conceptual frameworks (Burns & Grove 2005; Nieswiadomy 1993; Polit, Beck & Hungler 2001). A **theoretical framework** is based on propositional statements resulting from an existing theory, while a **conceptual framework** is one that the researcher has developed through identifying and defining concepts and proposing relationships between these concepts. Both frameworks interrelate concepts to create a specific way of looking at a particular phenomenon. By developing a framework within which ideas are organised, the researcher is able to show that the proposed study is a logical extension of current knowledge.

It is important that the 'fit' between the study variables and the selected theory is as tight as possible. The theory should apply to every step of the research process. To determine this, you need to familiarise yourself with a variety of theories, and then select the most applicable theory for your study. For example, a health care professional is concerned about incontinence in patients in a geriatric unit, and she wants to plan a study for modifying this. She studies a number of theories and thereafter selects a behavioural theory, namely, Skinner's reinforcement theory. She argues that incontinence is behaviour characterised by involuntary urination before the patient can get to the bathroom or be positioned on a bedpan. Skinner's theory suggests that behaviour can be modified with reinforcement. The health care professional believes that patients can be taught to control urination if effective reinforcers, such as special treats or other appropriate rewards, are applied. She is thus guided by Skinner's theory in the planning and conduct of her research to teach patients to control their urination.

Other theories that are frequently used as frameworks are Rosenstock's health belief model, Pender's health promotion model and Selye's stress theory, as well as the nursing theories of authorities such as Orem, King, Neumann, Leininger, and so on.

As a researcher, once you have identified a suitable conceptual framework, you should carefully evaluate its usefulness using the following types of questions:

- Is the theory appropriate to the research problem?
- Is it congruent with your beliefs and values?

In purely qualitative studies, the research problem may not be explained in terms of a theoretical or conceptual framework. Instead, the researcher may present a philosophical rationale or a central theoretical statement for studying the problem.

Development of theory

The first step in developing a theory is for you to become familiar with the structural and functional components. The **structural components** include assumptions, concepts, constructs and propositions, while the **functional components** consist of the domain concepts of the theory and how you should use them, that is, describe, explain, predict or control.

Assumptions are the basic principles that we accept on faith, or assume to be true without proof or verification (Polit, Beck & Hungler 2001). They determine the nature of concepts, definitions, purposes and relationships. They are the basic underlying truths from which theoretic reasoning proceeds.

Concepts are linguistic labels that we assign to objects or events. They have been described as the 'building blocks' of theories. Polit, Beck and Hungler (2001: 31) define them as "abstract characteristics of the subjects that are being studied". Concepts vary in level of abstraction. Highly abstract, complex concepts are, for example, self-esteem and coping. These are difficult to measure. Less abstract concepts, such as over- or underweight and blood loss, lend themselves more readily to empirical measurement. Generally, the more abstract and complex the concept, the more difficult it is for the researcher to derive valid and reliable empirical indicators.

Concepts are not defined or clarified in everyday usage. For example, when a patient describes him-/herself as 'sad', and you know what may be making them feel this way, the description may be sufficient for you to understand the patient. However, if you were to study the concept of sadness in depth, you would have to specify, clarify and define the emotion. Defining concepts allows consistency in the way we use such terms.

When a concept is clarified so that it is potentially observable, and in a form that is measurable, it is considered to be a **construct**. For example, a construct associated with the concept of pain might be physiological and psychological discomfort. As a rule, constructs are deliberately non-specific so that most health care professionals who deal with them will understand exactly what to measure, observe, control or look for in the real world. **Variables** are more precise and specific than concepts and constructs, and imply that the concept is defined so specifically that precise observations, and therefore measurements, can be accomplished. Figure 2.2 on the next page illustrates the links between concepts, constructs and variables.

Sometimes also referred to as 'relational statements', **propositions** are statements that suggest a specific relationship between two or more concepts or constructs. The nature of the relationship may take various forms. Some concepts may be related to other concepts in one way, or in several ways. Others stand alone and are unrelated to each other. Concepts may also be related negatively or positively.

Taken as a whole, propositions provide the substance and form of a theory. Figure 2.3 on the next page shows how a proposition could be developed.

	Example 1	Example 2	Level of abstraction
concept	pain	anxiety	abstract
construct	physiological and psychological discomfort resulting from internal or external stressors	emotional response	abstract
variable	the score obtained on the pain inventory self-test	palmar sweating	concrete

Figure 2.2 Concept – construct – variable

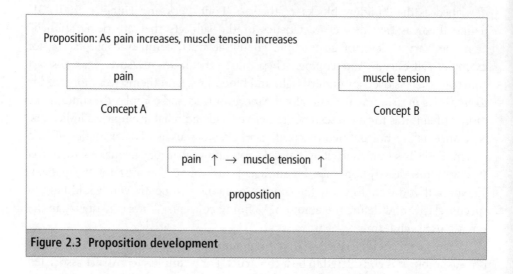

Proposition: As pain increases, muscle tension increases

pain

Concept A

muscle tension

Concept B

pain ↑ → muscle tension ↑

proposition

Figure 2.3 Proposition development

The development of theory requires a systematic process of enquiry. According to Chinn and Kramer (1991), there are various steps to the process. These need not be performed in the following order; in practice, there is flow of thought from one step to another and back as ideas are developed and refined:

1 Identify, select and clarify concepts.
2 Identify assumptions which form the grounding for the theory.
3 Clarify the context.
4 Develop relational statements through concept analysis, derivation or synthesis.
5 Test relational statements, and validate relationships.

There are numerous approaches to developing theory, most of which are shaped by logical positivists' views. Imagination and creativity are regarded as desirable characteristics in all approaches to theory building. Examples of those used in the health care sciences are induction, deduction and retroduction; theory derivation; model confirmation; borrowing and building with metaphors. Within these approaches specific theory-building strategies are explained and illustrated with examples from health sciences research. You may find the work of the following authors useful for further study on theory development: Chinn and Kramer (1991), Dubin (1978), Fawcett and Downs (1986), Meleis (1985), Moccia (1986), Moody (1990), and Walker and Avant (1988).

Testing of theory

Any health care sciences theory should be useful for the practice. Because it is an abstraction of reality, the theory must be tested to ensure that it represents the real world. The process of theory testing involves defining the concepts so that they can be measured, that is, developing operational definitions of the concepts, followed by devising propositions and hypotheses. The hypotheses are predictions about the manner in which variables would be related, if the theory were correct and useful. A theory is never tested directly. It is the hypotheses deduced from the theory that are subjected to scientific investigation.

The major focus of the testing process is comparison between observed outcomes of research and the relationships predicted by the hypotheses. Through this process the theory is continually subjected to potential disconfirmation. Repeated failure of research endeavours to disconfirm a theory results in increasing support for and acceptance of the theory.

Relationship between theory and research

It is worth reiterating that health sciences research and theory are interdependent and inseparable. Theory guides and generates ideas for research; research assesses the worth of existing theory and provides a foundation for new theory. Theories allow researchers to knit together observations and facts into an orderly system. They guide the researcher's understanding not only of the phenomena of interest but also of the reasons behind the occurrence of these phenomena. Theories help to stimulate research and the extension of knowledge by providing both direction and impetus.

Research plays an active role in the development of theory. It initiates, reformulates, deflects and clarifies theory. Evidently, theory and research are mutually beneficial. Moody (1990) describes the theory–research relationship as 'concatenated', which means that the two are linked within each series of events in the theory–research process. According to Stevens-Barnum (1990), the relationship is a recycling chain in which theory directs research, research corrects theory and corrected (or confirmed) theory directs further research.

However, such a relationship is not always evident in health sciences research. Health care professionals have been and continue to be criticised for producing numerous instances of isolated research that are difficult to integrate owing to the absence of a theoretical foundation. This retards the development of the health sciences in general. Therefore, we should regard the linking of theory and research as advantageous to the development of the health sciences. But it would be unreasonable for us to assert that research without any theoretical underpinning cannot make a contribution to science. In some cases, the research may be so pragmatic in nature that it does not *need* a theory to enhance its usefulness. Non-theoretical research has the potential to be linked to theory at a later date.

Summary

In this chapter we focused on the relationship between theory and research, referring to the various meanings attributed to theory and related terms in the health sciences research literature. Having provided and compared several definitions of the term 'theory', we outlined the different theories themselves, as described in the literature, and explored the definitions of terms related to theory. We paid attention to theory development and testing, and briefly discussed the steps used in both. Finally, we confirmed the interdependent nature of the relationship between theory and research.

Exercises

Complete these exercises:
1 Select a research article from the literature that describes a study guided by a conceptual or theoretical framework. Analyse how the framework influences the steps in the research process.
2 What would you say to try to convince a fellow researcher that it is advisable to use a framework – theoretical or conceptual – for a research project?
3 Analyse the research article that you selected in the first exercise and describe the paradigm that the researcher used.

3

Ethical considerations in the conduct of health sciences research

LEARNING OUTCOMES

On completion of this chapter, you should be able to demonstrate your understanding of

■ the basic ethical principles underlying protection of human subjects

■ the rights of human subjects that need to be recognised and protected by the researcher

■ the essential elements of an informed consent form, which complies with principles of research ethics and protects the rights of human subjects

■ the adequacy of a consent form

■ the factors that affect human subjects who are particularly vulnerable to risk in research

■ appropriate steps that the researcher must take in working with vulnerable groups

■ the risks and benefits associated with research procedures

■ steps that the researcher should take to safeguard the anonymity and confidentiality of research subjects

■ the role of institutional review boards and committees in the review of research proposals and reports

■ the ethical implications of a research report.

Introduction

A researcher is responsible for conducting research in an ethical manner. Failure to do so undermines the scientific process and may have negative consequences. To conduct research ethically, the researcher must

- carry out the research competently
- manage resources honestly
- acknowledge fairly those who contribute guidance or assistance
- communicate results accurately
- consider the consequences of the research for the field of study in particular, and for society in general.

While most of these concerns are relevant to all sciences, researchers involved in research with *human subjects* have special concerns – related to the protection of the rights of the human subjects. Unfortunately, researchers have not always paid attention to these concerns.

Codes of ethical research

As a result of the Nuremberg Trials, which were held to try members of the Nazi Party for their involvement in World War II and the Holocaust, there was a movement to protect human rights. The Nuremberg Code of 1947 was the first set of guidelines drawn up to protect the rights of research subjects. This Code mandated voluntary consent, justification of research for the good of society with appropriate balance of risk and benefit, adequate protection of subjects from risk or harm, the subject's right to withdraw from experimentation, and adequate scientific qualifications for researchers (Burns & Grove 2005: 177). The Code can be viewed on the internet at http://ohsr.od.nih.gov/nuremberg.php3.

Although this was an effective beginning, the Code omitted two major classes of research subjects: *children* and the *mentally incompetent* persons. Published in 1964, and amended in 1975, 1983 and 1989 by the World Health Organisation (WHO), the Declaration of Helsinki remedied the matter by including children, if parental permission is obtained, and mentally incompetent persons, if **proxy consent** – that is, consent from the closest family member – is obtained. The Declaration distinguishes between **therapeutic research**, which benefits the research subject, and **non-therapeutic research**, which does not directly benefit the subject, and sets stringent constraints on researchers undertaking the latter. The Declaration also reiterates the statements of the Nuremberg Code, and emphasises the importance of written consent (World Medical Association 1984). The Declaration was updated in 2004 and is available on the internet at http://ohsr.od.nih.gov/helsinki.php3.

The Nuremberg Code and the Declaration of Helsinki provide the foundation for numerous ethical research guidelines developed by government and professional organisations involved in the conduct of research on human subjects all over the world. In South Africa, the South African Medical Research Council (MRC) has developed guidelines called the 'Ethical Considerations in Medical Research'. These were first published in 1979, and a revised edition was published subsequently. The Human Sciences Research Council (HSRC) developed a Research Code (n.d.) for research in human sciences. In 1990, the then South African Nursing Association published 'Ethical Standards for Nursing Research'. Since then it has been updated by the Democratic Nursing Organisation of South Africa in 1998 and again in 2005. (See Annexure A).

While ethical principles relating to subject protection play a primary role in these documents, there are other important principles as well. These deal with sensitive issues such as honesty and integrity in conducting research, the responsibilities of the researcher, sharing and utilising data, truthful reporting of results and assigning authorship on scientific publications describing the research. Unethical research is rarely intentional, but it often occurs when the rights of participants are in conflict with the demands of the research problems (Polit, Beck & Hungler 2001). For example, participants may experience side-effects, such as discomfort, in a trial of a drug that may be a 'medical breakthrough'. In order to avoid this, the researcher needs to base his/her research on ethical principles from the start, and ensure that he/she adheres to these principles through the entire process.

Fundamental ethical principles

There are three fundamental ethical principles that guide researchers: respect for persons, beneficence and justice. These principles are based on the human rights that need to be protected in research, namely, the right to self-determination, to privacy, to anonymity and confidentiality, to fair treatment and to being protected from discomfort and harm. Table 3.1 summarises these rights and the factors involved.

Table 3.1 Human rights to be protected in research

Rights	Unethical approach	Affected subjects
Right to self-determination	Violation of the right to self-determination	All subjects
	Persons with diminished autonomy	Legally and mentally incompetent subjects Adults Terminally ill subjects Subjects confined to institutions

31

Rights	Unethical approach	Affected subjects
Right to privacy	Violation of privacy	All subjects
Right to anonymity and confidentiality	Using real names	All subjects
Right to fair treatment	Unfair selection and treatment of subjects	All subjects
Right to protection from discomfort and harm	No anticipated effects Temporary discomfort Unusual levels of temporary discomfort Risk of permanent damage Certainty of permanent damage	All subjects

Source: Adapted from Burns and Grove (2005).

We will now explore the ethical principles in more detail.

Principle of respect for persons

This principle involves three convictions:

1 Individuals are autonomous, that is, they have the right to **self-determination**. This implies that an individual has the right to decide whether or not to participate in a study, without the risk of penalty or prejudicial treatment. In addition, he/she has the right to withdraw from the study at any time, to refuse to give information or to ask for clarification about the purpose of the study. The researcher must respect this right by avoiding using any form of coercion.

2 Individuals with diminished autonomy require **protection**. This group includes children, the mentally impaired, patients who are unconscious and patients who are institutionalised.

Principle of beneficence

To adhere to this principle, the researcher needs to secure the well-being of the subject, who has a **right to protection from discomfort and harm** – be it physical, emotional, spiritual, economical, social or legal. If the research problem involves a potentially harmful intervention, it may have to be abandoned or restated to allow investigation in an ethical environment. For example, it would be unethical for a researcher to manipulate the amount of smoking and alcohol drinking in a pregnant subject in order to observe the effects of these substances on the baby. Before the study is allowed to take place, the review committee should pose this question: Can the information be found from any other source or by means of any research method other than the one in which there is anticipated direct harm to the subject?

Although qualitative research is often regarded as 'non-invasive' because it involves neither intervention nor treatment, qualitative researchers nevertheless enter the participants' lives. By its very nature, qualitative enquiry risks exploring as yet unresolved issues, which can upset the participants. A researcher should always use good clinical judgement to manage each interview in this type of study, and should organise support from the primary caregivers before leaving the participant to him-/ herself (Munhall 2001). The researcher must try to avoid harming participants, and can do this by carefully structuring the questions and monitoring the participants for any sign of distress. Should this occur, the researcher needs to facilitate debriefing by giving participants the opportunity to ask questions or air complaints, and, if necessary, by referring them for counselling (Polit, Beck & Hungler 2001).

As researchers, we must always remember that we "are guests in the private spaces of the world. [Our] manners should be good and [our] code of ethics strict" (Stake 2003: 154).

Principle of justice

This principle includes the subjects' **right to fair selection and treatment**. The researcher must select with fairness the study population in general, and the subjects in particular. He/she should select the subjects for reasons directly related to the study problem, and not because they are readily available or can be easily manipulated. Nor should the researcher's choice be motivated by a desire for the subjects to receive the specific benefits that the study might offer. Subjects should also be treated fairly – the researcher must respect any agreements that he/she made with the subjects. If data collection must be done in an interview situation, the researcher should always be punctual, and should terminate the process at the agreed time. The researcher must also remember to provide any incentive that he/she promised, at the start of the study.

The researcher must also respect the subjects' **right to privacy**. The subject has the right to determine the extent to which, and the general circumstances under which, his/her private information will be shared with or withheld from others, in contrast to the patient–doctor relationship, in which the doctor is legally bound not to tell anyone the details of the patient's case. Such information includes the subject's attitudes, beliefs, behaviour, opinions and medical records. A researcher who *gathers* data from subjects without their knowledge – by taping conversations, observing through one-way mirrors and using hidden cameras and microphones – invades the privacy of the subjects. Invasion also occurs when the researcher *shares* private information without the subjects' knowledge or against his/her will.

In order to respect the subject's right to privacy, the researcher should refrain from what is called 'covert data collection', which entails the use of questions such as the following:

- Do you use drugs?
- Are you gay?
- What are your sexual activities?
- Were you abused as a child?

A subject who agrees to participate in research has a right to expect that the information collected from or about him/her will remain private. This can be ensured through either anonymity or confidentiality procedures.

'Anonymity' literally means namelessness. The **process of ensuring anonymity** refers to the researcher's act of keeping the subjects' identities a secret with regard to their participation in the research study. In fact, it is preferable that even the researcher should not be able to link a subject with his/her data. For example, by distributing questionnaires and requiring that they be returned without any identifying details, the researcher ensures that the subjects' responses remain anonymous. If the results of the study are to be published, the researcher must assure the subjects of the safeguards that he/she has put in place to protect their identities. This is particularly important when there are few subjects in the study and the research setting is easily identifiable.

Research that is designed so that data are collected only once presents few problems in terms of anonymity. When data are collected in one sitting, the use of names is unnecessary as there will be only one set of responses (even if there is more than one subject). By contrast, research that is designed to compare individual performance over time presents a challenge to the researcher with regard to ensuring participant anonymity. The researcher may have to follow up an issue and would need a list of participants' names so that he/she can contact them at a later date. This obviously increases the potential for the subjects' right to anonymity to be violated. In such a case, as well as in other cases where anonymity is impossible, the researcher must be particularly careful in clarifying or explaining the situation to the subjects, and implementing appropriate confidentiality procedures.

In situations such as focus group interviews or even individual interviews, absolute anonymity is not possible. Nevertheless, the researcher can *process* the data anonymously. When publishing case studies, owing to the detailed nature of the descriptions, the researcher may have to change some of the information in such a manner that the participants are not recognised. It is quite common, for example, for a person's name and age to be changed, or for the name of a company to be altered, as long as this does not interfere with the focus of the case study itself.

The researcher can use any of the following mechanisms to ensure anonymity:

- Provide each participant with a number or code name, or have him/her devise his/her own code.

- Use the code names when discussing data.
- Keep the master list of participants' names and matching code numbers in a safe place.
- Destroy the list of real names.

The **process of ensuring confidentiality** refers to the researcher's responsibility to prevent all data gathered during the study from being divulged or made available to any other person. The exception to this is if the information is published for the benefit of other researchers or scientists in the field, in which case the researcher must keep the subjects informed and assure them that he/she will protect their anonymity. Data in the form of responses to questionnaires, video and audio tape interviews, and transcriptions thereof, should be kept in a secure place, such as a safe.

A breach of confidentiality occurs when a researcher allows an unauthorised person to gain access to the study data, or when he/she accidentally or otherwise reveals the subjects' identities in reporting or publishing the research findings. It may happen that the institution from which the researcher plans to collect the data requests access to the information, or family members or close friends express the desire to see data that the researcher has collected on a specific subject. Furthermore, other researchers may request the data to use in their own research. It is important that the researcher plans ahead for such possibilities, and ensures that they are taken into account when he/she seeks the subject's informed consent.

Procedures and mechanisms for protecting human rights

There are various procedures and mechanisms that a researcher can use in the course of a study to ensure that the abovementioned rights of the subjects are protected. We will now explore them in detail.

Informed consent

The ethical principles of voluntary participation and protecting the participants from harm are formalised in the concept of 'informed consent' (Babbie & Mouton 2001). Informed consent has three major elements:

1　The type of information needed from the research subject.
2　The degree of understanding that the subject must have in order to give consent.
3　The fact that the subject has the choice of whether or not to give consent.

Information

In order to obtain the subject's consent, the researcher must provide him/her with comprehensive and clear information regarding his/her participation in the study.

The researcher can provide the information

- in **written form** – the researcher gives the necessary information to the subject in writing
- in **verbal form** – the researcher discusses the proposed research project with the subject
- in **taped form**, that is, audio or video recording – the researcher records the necessary information on audio or video tape and gives the tape to or watch the subject to listen to either immediately or at home at a later stage.

The researcher must select the appropriate method after careful consideration of the potential participant's cognitive ability – is he/she highly literate, literate, barely literate or illiterate? – and developmental level – what is the best way to present the information? is he/she a child or an adult?

There is no strict format for the written consent, though it must include the following information:

- The title of the research project.
- An introduction to the research activities, that is, extending the invitation for the subject to participate in the study.
- The researcher's title and position. This enhances the credibility of the study.
- The purpose of the project, including the long-term purpose.
- The selection of the study population and the sample. This indicates the population to be studied, as well as how and why they were selected.
- An explanation of methods and procedures by which data will be collected.
- A description of any risks and discomfort (be it physical, psychological, emotional, economic or social) involved, as well as benefits.
- A suggestion of alternative treatment, when the study involves an intervention or treatment.
- Confirmation of anonymity and confidentiality.
- The voluntary nature of participation. The subject must sign a non-coercive disclaimer, which is a statement that his/her participation is voluntary and that refusal to participate will not involve any penalty or loss of benefits, such as routine care or treatment. The subject must be made aware that he/she may withdraw at any time, without risk to his/her well-being or care.
- Consent to incomplete disclosure. When full disclosure could harm the validity of the study, the subject should know that the researcher is withholding some of the information deliberately. We discuss this further below.
- The offer of the researcher to answer any questions that the subject may pose.
- The name of a contact person, in case a participant needs to talk to someone regarding his/her participation.

▓ A clearly delineated space for the signatures of the researcher and the research participant as well as a witness.

Figure 3.1 on the next page is an example of an informed consent form.

Understanding, or comprehension

As well as simply receiving the abovementioned information, the subject must understand that information. Therefore, it should be in the subject's own language, at his/her level of understanding and in his/her vocabulary, not in technical language or professional jargon.

The researcher can take steps to determine whether the subject understands the information, for example, by asking him/her questions directly related to the information that he/she has received.

Choice

The researcher is responsible for ensuring that the subject invited to participate in the study is not unduly influenced to participate, or coerced, which is that he/she is made to feel that he/she must participate. For example, a researcher could try to force the subject to participate by threatening to withhold the benefits if he/she does not participate. This would be unethical. A prospective subject has to decide voluntarily whether or not to participate in a study, and must be given time to do so. He/she must feel confident that refusal to participate will not prejudice him/her in any way.

Voluntary consent is obtained only once the subject has demonstrated a clear understanding of the essential information provided in the informed consent form.

Most of the procedures that need informed consent on the part of the subject are based on experimental studies. In this case, the researcher must obtain the subject's informed consent at the start. In the case of qualitative research, informed consent is an *ongoing* process. As the study develops, the researcher should re-obtain the subject's informed consent as unexpected events may occur, or new research questions could emerge. The situation implies that the researcher must "ask participants for permission to change [the] first agreement' (Munhall 2001: 544). The act of re-obtainment is known as **process consent**.

Issues relating to informed consent

Although most researchers endorse the subject's rights to self-determination and informed consent, there are circumstances that make these standards difficult to uphold in practice.

TITLE: EATING PATTERNS SUCCESSFUL DIETERS USE TO MAINTAIN WEIGHT LOSS

INVESTIGATOR: WENDY CHABOYER
                              RN. MN

In response to your reply to the advertisement in the *Morning Star* for successful dieters, I am herewith inviting you to participate in a research study on successful dieters. The purpose of the research is to see if there are any common features in the personal histories of successful dieters (weight losers) that can be shared with unsuccessful weight losers. Although this study will not benefit you directly, the information obtained may help those who have trouble in losing weight and maintaining weight loss to hear how you (and other successful dieters) were able to do it.

purpose

potential benefit

As far as I can tell, there should be no risks or discomforts to you in sharing your own story. Your participation will mean that you will meet with me once for an audio-taped interview lasting one to one-and-a-half hours. You will be requested to provide a photograph of yourself when overweight or a piece of clothing you may have saved, and I will ask you to weigh yourself on my calibrated scale and to let me measure your height.

risks

time commitment

I will keep a record of who has participated in this study, and I will keep the tapes of our interviews, together with a transcription of those tapes. Your name will not be on the tape or on the transcription of those tapes, so that data will not be linked with your name. All data will be stored in a secure place and no one except the reach team will have access to your interview. Your identity will not be revealed when the study is reported or published.

explanation of procedures
anonymity
confidentiality

If you have any questions about the study or about participating in the study, please feel free to ask me (Wendy Chaboyer). You may call me at (001) 111 111 (work) or (222) 999 999 (home).

offer to answer questions

Your participation in this study is totally voluntary: you are under no obligation to participate. You have the right to withdraw at any time if you care to, without repercussion or penalty, even in the middle of the interview.

voluntary consent
option to withdraw

The study and its procedures have been approved by the appropriate people and research committees of Gauteng University.

(Board or Committee approval)

I have discussed the above points with the subject. It is my opinion that the subject understands the risks, benefits and obligations involved in participating in this project.

_____   _____
          Investigator   Date

I understand that my participation is voluntary and that I may refuse to participate or withdraw my consent and stop taking part at any time without penalty.

I hereby freely consent to take part in this research project.

_____   _____   _____
   Signature of witness   Signature of subject   Date

Figure 3.1 An example of an informed consent form

One of the issues concerns certain people's inability to make well-informed decisions. Vulnerable people, for example those who are mentally challenged, may be incapable of giving full informed consent. In the case of children and mentally challenged people, the researcher must obtain a proxy consent, as we explained earlier in this chapter. A pregnant woman and the unborn baby are extremely vulnerable. In this case, the researcher should make absolutely sure that the risk is extremely low in comparison to the possible benefit.

In certain situations the researcher cannot tell the subject about every aspect of a research procedure as this could negate the effect of the treatment. For example, the reaction of a group of health sciences students to a crisis situation will be artificial if the group knows that the crisis is being staged by the researcher in order to investigate the nature of their reaction. In this case the researcher may withhold information from the participants or even provide them with false information. This means that the researcher is using deception.

Some researchers argue that the use of deception is never justified. Others believe that if the study involves minimal risk to subjects, if there are anticipated benefits to science and society, and if there are no other research alternatives to obtain the information, then the deception may be justified. When using deception, the researcher must inform the subjects of the reasons for the deception (without going into detail), discuss with them any misconceptions they may have about the research, and in general attempt to remove any harmful effects of the deception. This process is called **debriefing**.

The risk–benefit ratio

Before beginning the study, researchers and reviewers of research must examine the ratio between the benefits and risks involved. The benefits are the positive values that the research provides, for example the study's potential contribution to knowledge, practical value to society and benefit to the subject. Risk refers to the possibility that the participant may be harmed during the research. As in most aspects of daily life, all research involves a certain amount of risk.

The general guideline is that the risk should not exceed the potential benefits to be gained by the study. When the risk is high, the researcher must make every effort to reduce it and to maximise the benefits. Should the risk outweigh the benefits of the study, the study should not be undertaken.

Major potential *benefits* include the following:
- Increased knowledge about health care practice or the subject's condition.
- Improvement in the subject's understanding of health care delivery.
- Enhanced self-esteem in the subject as a result of the special attention that he/she has been given.

- Subject's rapid recovery from illness.
- Improvement in health care delivery to the public.
- Improved assessment of health needs.
- Increased understanding of preventive health measures.

Major potential *risks* include the following:
- Physical harm to the subject in the form of unanticipated side-effects. In the case of serious unanticipated side-effects, the study should be stopped immediately and reported to the relevant ethics committee.
- Physical discomfort, fatigue or boredom on the part of the subject.
- Psychological or emotional distress in the subject, resulting from self-disclosure, introspection, fear of the unknown or fear of repercussions.
- Loss of privacy.
- Loss of time.
- Financial costs.

The obligation to make sure that the benefits outweigh the risks of the study is not only the responsibility of the researcher – other professionals and society are also accountable. Professionals must be members of research boards and committees to ensure the conduct of ethical research, and society needs to be concerned about the entire enterprise of research and about the protection of subjects from harm (Burns & Grove 2005).

Scientific honesty and other responsibilities

In addition to respecting the rights of the subject, the researcher must demonstrate respect for the scientific community by protecting the integrity of scientific knowledge. As we mention above, the researcher has ethical responsibilities associated with the conduct and reporting of the research. He/she must be competent, accurate and, above all, honest in everything that he/she does.

In order to be honest, the researcher must *avoid* the following activities:
- **Fabrication, falsification or forging.** For example, the researcher invents information, or makes a report that does not reflect what he/she actually did.
- **Manipulation of design and methods.** For example, the researcher plans the design and data-collection methods so that the results will support his/her point of view.
- **Selective retainment and/or manipulation of data.** For example, the researcher chooses only the data that will support his/her point of view and discards the rest, or manipulates the data to reflect his/her viewpoint.
- **Plagiarism.** For example, the researcher presents as his/her own the work or ideas of someone else.

- **Irresponsible collaboration.** For example, as a member of a research team, the researcher participates inappropriately or does not fulfil his/her responsibility as a co-author of the report (Struwig & Stead 2001).

It is also important for the researcher to manage resources, be they financial, human or material, in an effective, efficient and economical manner. Research that is poorly planned and conducted is likely to be ineffective and inefficient, and wastes the time and effort of the researcher and of the subjects. Such conduct is unethical. Furthermore, the researcher must obtain permission to conduct the study from the relevant authorities, employers and owners of the institutions, premises or materials which he/she intends using for the research.

Today, ethics in internet research has become a crucial issue for researchers. Researchers need to ensure that data drawn from the internet is reliable and valid. This is often difficult owing to a lack of information about the credibility of the website concerned. Researchers also use the internet as a means of reaching and collecting information from their subjects. There are problems associated with this method too. Researchers may not be aware of the subjects' circumstances and may misinterpret the results. Not everyone has access to a computer, a fact which may lead to selection bias. Moreover, confidentiality and privacy can be violated. The transmission of information and the storage of questionnaires in particular are problematic – hackers can access the researchers' computers and read the data.

Many of these issues are currently under investigation. Researchers need to bear them in mind, and develop strategies to protect participants (Struwig & Stead 2001).

Ethics review boards and committees

In addition to research codes or ethical guidelines (an example of which we provide in Annexure A), most institutions have set up independent committees to review proposed research, and to examine and monitor the ethical standards of ongoing research. These committees are called 'institutional review boards' (IRBs), 'ethics committees' or 'research committees'. Researchers must submit their research proposals along with the necessary consent forms to the appropriate committee for review, prior to beginning the research project. Whether they are undergraduates performing a research project in order to meet course requirements, professionals undertaking research or doctoral students doing research with the goal of publishing their findings in a scientific journal, researchers must be aware of the ethical rules and regulations governing research at their institution, and must have ethical clearance for their studies before they embark on data collection.

Remember that as a researcher you are not the best person to evaluate the ethical value of your study. You should turn to the ethics committee of your institution for guidance and advice.

Role of ethics review boards and committees

The submission of the research proposal for review by a committee or board is a policy that protects the researcher and the research subjects. The members of the committee or board will consider every aspect of the proposed research, including the ethical aspects that we discuss above. The members may refuse permission for the researcher to carry out the study, or they may recommend changes to the research proposal if they are not satisfied that it is in accordance with the established scientific and ethical guidelines.

In the USA, many research studies are exempted from review (Polit, Beck & Hungler 2001), which means that they do not need to be reviewed before they can take place. Usually, this is if they have no apparent risks for the research subject. For example, these are studies dealing with normal educational practices; surveys, interviews or observations of public behaviour that do not identify subjects or place them at risk, or that do not involve sensitive behaviour; and those that make use of publicly available data, such as artefacts, photographs and historical documents. Even if studies are exempt, however, the responsibility of the researcher to protect the subjects of the study does not change.

Evaluation of the ethical elements of a research proposal or report

As a researcher you may be called upon to serve on a research committee or review board, or to assess the research proposals or reports of peers. In the same way that a research proposal must be ethically acceptable to be approved, ethical implications are also highly important if you are considering adopting research findings in practice. An ethical committee's checklist is an excellent guide that you can use when you must review a report. Many textbooks on health care sciences research also provide checklists. Alternatively, you can compile a checklist yourself.

However, the reports frequently do not provide detailed information regarding the degree to which the researcher adhered to the necessary ethical principles, because of space limitations in professional journals – where these reports are most likely to be made available. But even without such a detailed description, there are various factors of the report that you can evaluate from an ethical point of view. You can apply the following questions to the report:

- Is the research problem significant?
- Is the design scientifically sound?
- Is the research designed to maximise the benefits to the subjects and minimise the risks?
- Are the appropriate steps taken not to physically harm or psychologically distress the subjects?
- Is the selection of subjects ethically appropriate?

- Is there evidence of voluntary informed consent? If not, is there a valid and justifiable reason?
- Has informed consent been given by the legal guardian or representative of a subject who is incapable of giving his/her own consent?
- Is there evidence of deception?
- Are appropriate steps taken to safeguard the privacy of the subject?

Summary

In this chapter, we presented in detail the need for professional ethical guidelines in conducting health care research. We explored the rights of the subjects as well as the ways in which researchers can protect those rights. This includes how subjects are selected and invited to participate in the study, what information they must be given, what choice they have, how confidentiality and anonymity will be maintained, what risks have been identified and how to minimise them while maximising the benefits. We considered scientific honesty. The chapter closed with a discussion of the role of ethics review boards and committees and provided a set of guidelines that a member of such a board or committee can use to evaluate the ethical implications of a research report.

Exercises

Complete these exercises:

1 A researcher plans a study to determine third-year students' behaviour in a crisis situation. She wants to observe reactions to crisis as these might occur naturally. Thus, she decides not to tell the students the exact nature of the study. Each student is instructed to measure the blood pressure of a patient as part of the patient's continuous assessment. The patient, who is a volunteer and has been briefed by the researcher, simulates an epileptic fit while the blood pressure is being taken. A research assistant observes the timeliness and appropriateness of the students' responses through a one-way mirror. Immediately afterwards the students are debriefed and paid R10 for their participation.

   a) Discuss the ethical implications of conducting this study with emphasis on the risk–benefit ratio, and on the subjects' rights to self-determination and privacy. Was there a valid and justifiable reason for the researcher not obtaining informed consent?

   b) What type of subjects review would be appropriate for this study?

   c) Describe any debriefing that this study should include.

2 A researcher plans to investigate the efficacy of three alternative methods for alleviating sunburn. Develop a summary describing the key aspects of the study that the researcher should present to the subjects when seeking their consent.

Here are some website addresses that you may find useful:

Medical Research Council: http://www.mrc.ac.za
National Research Foundation: http://www.nrf.ac.za
American Nurses Association Code of Ethics for Nurses:
    http://www.ana.org/ethic/chcode.htm
International Council for Nurses: http://www.icn.ch
International Confederation of Midwives: http://www.internationalmidwives.org

APPENDIX A
Standards for nursing research

ETHICAL STANDARDS FOR NURSE RESEARCHERS
Reproduced with permission of the Democratic Nursing Organisation of
South Africa (DENOSA).

DENOSA believes that the following standards should be adhered to:
1. Nursing research is planned and executed in a way that will foster good, ethical research, justice, beneficence and exclude harm/exploitation of participants in accordance with certain criteria.
2. The right to self-determination by the participant(s) in the research project is ensured by the researcher in accordance with certain criteria.
3. Confidentiality and anonymity is ensured in accordance with certain criteria.
4. Quality research is ensured in accordance with certain criteria.

First approved August, 1998
Updated October, 2005

1.   INTRODUCTION
The ethical standards for nurse researchers serve as a framework for nurses conducting and participating in research. The standards also serve as criteria against which nurses, as advocates for their patients, can judge proposed research in which their patients will be study subjects, as well as to evaluate and account for the ethical standards in nursing research.

These standards refer primarily to clinical research, but apply equally to all nursing research and include the rights and responsibilities of all the role players in research.

2.   ETHICAL STANDARDS
2.1   **Nursing research is planned and executed in a way which will foster good, ethical research, justice, beneficence and exclude harm/exploitation of participants in accordance with the following criteria:**
2.1.1   Assessment of possible physical or psychological or emotional discomfort/harm is conducted by the researcher prior to the commencement of the research project.
2.1.2   Any possible known identified discomfort/harm for the participant(s) is explained during the process of obtaining informed consent.
2.1.3   Any possible identified discomfort/harm shall not exceed that which could be encountered in daily life experience by the participant or as part of his/her illness at that stage.
2.1.4   Any possible identified discomfort/harm shall cease with the termination of the research project.
2.1.5   The negative effects of unavoidable discomfort/distress experienced by the participant after completion of the participation, are only acceptable if the benefits outweigh these negative/unavoidable effects and with informed consent of the participant.
2.1.6   Fair and equal treatment of participants during a clinical trial all other research is ensured by equalization of advantages after completion of the clinical trial.
2.1.7   There is no victimization or loss of benefits of a participant that refuses to participate in the research, or has withdrawn during the participation.
2.1.8   Approval is obtained from the relevant Research Ethics Committee(s) and the Committee receives notice of any on/with final completion of study.
2.1.9   A contact person is made available to participants for questions regarding the research project.

2.2   The right to self-determination by the participant(s) in the research project is ensured by the researcher in accordance with the following criteria:

2.2.1   Informed consent is obtained by the researcher.

2.2.2   Informed consent is obtained from the relevant authority.

2.2.3   Informed consent is obtained from the relevant participant(s).

2.2.4   The legal requirements in terms (of) minor/participant unable to give informed consent are adhered to.

2.2.5   Informed consent is obtained from captive group(s) involved in a dependent relationship with the researcher, by the way of procedures approved by the peer group.

2.2.6   Informed consent is obtained from the field workers/collectors of data.

2.2.7   Research without patient consent is only executed during observational research totally without risk, or innocuous research involving comprehension.

2.2.8   The true purpose of the research without patient consent is declared to the patients as soon as possible.

2.2.9   Transparency is upheld in terms of the objectives of the research, type of data to be collected, method of data collection and possible benefit(s) to the authority and participant(s).

2.2.10   Any financial liability (by both the researcher, participant and funder) is adhered to according to an agreement.

2.3   Confidentiality and anonymity is ensured in accordance with the following criteria:

2.3.1   Protection of the participant's(s) identity.

2.3.2   The researcher ensures privacy, worth and dignity of the participant(s).

2.3.3   The researcher ensures that no linking between the individual identity of participant(s) or oganisation(s) to the research data can be made.

2.4   Quality research is ensured in accordance with the following criteria:

2.4.1   The researcher(s) has the liability (knowledge, skills and attitude) to execute the research process (researcher includes the supervisor/mentor).

2.4.2   The researcher(s) adheres to the standards of planning, implementation, evaluation and reporting of research.

2.4.3   The researcher conforms to the principles of sampling in a rigid and trustworthy manner.

2.4.4   The researcher demonstrates integrity (honesty, to act in good faith, adherence to pre-determined agreements) throughout the process.

2.4.5   The researcher ensures that the process and results are trustworthy/valid.

2.4.6 Thorough and complete documentation of the research process and results to enable a trustworthy audit trail (retrospective auditing).

2.4.7 The researcher(s) accepts and demonstrats accountability for the research process and results.

2.4.8 The researcher is accountable for the appropriate dissemination of the results and recommendations.

2.4.9 The research is meaningful and contributes to the improvement of nursing practice (clinical, educational, ethical and managerial).

3. **DENOSA POSITION**

DENOSA is of the opinion that these four ethical standards should be adhered to in all research projects in order to ensure that all rights and responsibilities of the various role players are upheld.

Resources

Babbie, E & Mouton, J. 2002. *The practice of social research. South African Edition.* Cape Town: Oxford University Press.

Consultation with the nursing and midwifery profession during 2005.

De Vos, AS (ed). 2002. *Research at grass roots. For the social sciences and human service professions.* Second edition. Pretoria: Van Schaik.

International Council of Nurses. 1996. *Ethical Guidelines for Nursing Research.* Geneva: ICN.

Muller, ME. 2002: *Nursing Dynamics.* Third edition. Johannesburg: Heinemann.

Neuman, WL. 2003. *Social research methods. Qualitative and quantitative approaches.* Fifth edition. USA: Pearson Education.

Polit, DF & Beck, CT. 2006. *Essentials of nursing research. Methods, appraisal and utilization.* Sixth edition. Philadelphia: Lippincott.

South African Medical Research Council, 2002. *Revised guidelines for medical research.* Tygerberg MRC.

4 An overview of the research process

LEARNING OUTCOMES

On completion of this chapter, you should be able to demonstrate your understanding of

- the major phases of the research process
- the steps of the research process that are likely to occur in each phase
- a practical model of the research process in health sciences.

Introduction

In this chapter we present a general overview of the research process. In later chapters we will discuss each phase and step in greater detail. Note that the research process we present here is a *model*; it gives an idealised representation of reality. By contrast, in reality, the flow of activities we present in chronological order will not always follow neatly one after the other, with each phase being complete before the next begins. Some phases may occur concurrently, or the researcher may work on more than one step at a time. Sometimes the researcher may omit a step and come back to it later.

In every case, however, there should be a general flow of activities that is typical of scientific investigation; in other words, the researcher should address the flow of activities in an orderly and systematic manner, even if he/she varies the order itself slightly. Therefore, a model of the research process provides a useful overview and serves as an effective guide.

The research process

Research is a process that begins with a problem and ends with the problem either resolved or addressed. Research is rarely conclusive; rather, it takes the form of a spiral, as it tends to engender new problems or areas of exploration. Research stimulates further research and cannot be seen as a once-off, linear, static act.

Broadly speaking, the framework for the research process consists of four interactive phases:

1 The **conceptual phase**, also called the 'thinking' or 'planning phase'. The standard element in this phase is the research *problem*.
2 The **empirical phase**, also called the 'doing phase'. The standard element in this phase is the research *design*.
3 The **interpretive phase**, or the phase where the researcher engages with the meaning of the study. The standard element in this phase is the *empirical evidence*.
4 The **communication phase**, or the phase of writing the research report. The standard element in this phase is the set of *conclusions*.

Each phase may be divided into various steps, which depend on the purpose of the study as well as on the research approach and design. In the literature, there is a difference of opinion as to the actual number of steps identified as necessary to the research process. While the number of steps varies from 8 to 17, the important issue is that the research process must flow logically and scientifically to address the identified problem.

We prefer a model with 11 steps, as we outline in Table 4.1. As a researcher, you may find it necessary to adapt this model to the specific needs of your research project. This is acceptable, provided that you clearly motivate any change, and that you thoroughly consider and record the implications of such a change on the research process as a whole and the subjects in particular.

You must view the steps in Table 4.1 as being interdependent and interrelated. This may seem confusing at first, but it often merely reflects the varying amounts of detail included, and the different ways of categorising specific activities associated with research.

You also need to be aware of the distinction between differing accounts in the literature, and of how this relates to the qualitative and quantitative research approaches. The steps in Table 4.1 are suitable for a quantitative approach. Using a qualitative approach, the researcher could omit Step 4 of the framework, as this type of research requires him/her to gather data with as open a mind as possible. The researcher cannot begin with a focused question, nor is he/she concerned with testing a hypothesis. Step 7 would also not be feasible in most qualitative research and therefore could be omitted.

Table 4.1 Steps in the research process	
1 Identify the problem or research question 2 Determine the purpose of the study 3 Search and review the literature relating to the question and develop a framework 4 Define and refine the research question or formulate a research hypothesis 5 Select the research method and determine the design of the study 6 Specify the group of subjects to be studied	PHASE 1
7 Conduct a 'dummy' run, or pilot study, of the research 8 Collect the data	PHASE 2
9 Analyse the data 10 Interpret the results	PHASE 3
11 Communicate the research findings	PHASE 4

Major phases and steps in the research process

Phase 1: The conceptual phase

Research normally begins with Phase 1, which typically involves activities with a strong conceptual element. 'Conceptualisation' refers to the process of developing and refining abstract ideas. During this phase, the researcher categorises and labels his/her impressions. Thus, the activities include thinking, reading, rethinking, theorising, making decisions, and reviewing ideas with colleagues, research partners or mentors. The researcher also needs to draw on the skills and abilities of creativity, analysis and insight, as well as on the firm grounding of existing research on the topic of interest.

Step 1: Identify the problem or research question

A research project begins with a problem or question. To a degree, good research depends on good questions. Without a workable, significant topic, the most carefully and skilfully designed research project is of little value. Problems or questions may come from various sources such as personal experience, issues considered important by communities or organisations, and clinical situations in health care, the literature or theories. Researchers generally proceed from the selection of a broad topic area to the development of a set of specific questions.

A clear, researchable question is the key to the researcher's decisions about the research design, data collection and analysis.

Step 2: Determine the purpose of the study

The research purpose is generated from the problem; it identifies the specific aim or goal of the study. It also describes the scope of the research effort, and specifies the information that needs to be addressed by the research process. Whereas the problem addresses the topic to be studied, the purpose gives the reason for the study. The researcher may wish to identify, describe, investigate, explain or predict a solution to the problem, or to evaluate a practice or programme, or to develop an instrument.

Step 3: Review the related literature

The literature review generates a picture of what is known and not known about the research problem. It is essential for the researcher to conduct a literature review in order to locate existing similar or related studies that can serve as a basis for the study at hand. The literature review will also help the researcher to develop a theoretical or conceptual framework for the study, as well as the relevant study methods and instruments or tools with which to measure the study variables.

The review should be comprehensive; it must cover all relevant research and supporting documents in print, such as textbooks, reports, journal articles, theses, dissertations, periodical and citation indexes, and other indexes in websites on the internet. A single visit to the library is insufficient; a thorough review of the related literature requires a great deal of time and effort. Computer-generated searches can assist tremendously with this step, but they should not totally replace the hard copy textual investigations of a dedicated researcher.

Occasionally, the initial review of the literature may *precede* the identification of the problem as, through reading, the researcher's conceptual insights and ideas regarding possible topics, and even approaches or techniques, may be stimulated.

Step 4: Define and refine the research question or formulate a research hypothesis

In this step, the researcher must construct the research problem in a way that facilitates further research. The problem should be made measurable, or should generate or refine essential knowledge. This involves the researcher moving from a broad, abstractly stated problem and general purpose to specific objectives, questions or hypotheses. These should provide direction and a specific focus, and must be stated clearly. For example, the researcher may state an objective such as: 'The purpose is to identify the five most frequently expressed needs of family members in intensive care waiting rooms'. Or he/she could ask: 'What are the characteristics of mothers who have difficulty bonding with their newborn babies?'. In this case, the researcher may have found information suggesting that ignorance affects maternal bonding with newborns. The hypothesis could be: 'First-time mothers who attend childbirth classes will demonstrate bonding with their newborn babies earlier than will mothers who do not attend the classes'.

Step 5: Select the research method and determine the design of the study

In this step, the researcher must design the study. The choice of design depends on the researcher's expertise, on the problem and purpose of the study, and on the researcher's desire to generalise the findings. Therefore, the researcher needs to make the following decisions by asking him-/herself certain questions:

- **Approach.** Which research approach – for example, quantitative or qualitative – will best answer the research question and meet the objectives? Which design is best – for example, a descriptive design, a case study, an experiment, an ethnographic study, a phenomenological study or a historical study? Considerations must include permission that might be required, ethical dilemmas that could occur, the timing of each step of the project, and defining of terminology.
- **Instrument.** What procedure should be used to gather the data? Should one or more tools be used to collect data? Should an existing tool be used, or one that has already been tested? What instrument would yield the most significant information? Will the tool yield reliable and valid information? What type of data should the instrument generate – for example, numerical or non-numerical?
- **Data-collection procedure (protocol).** Which are the various procedures for collecting the information, and what are the advantages and disadvantages of each? What are the time and financial constraints with regard to, for example, travel and actual collection of data?
- **Data analysis plan.** What is to be done with the data once it has been gathered?
- **Population and sample.** Who will constitute the population? Which population is accessible and can be best represented in the study? Which criteria are to be used in the selection of the sample, and in the decision concerning size of the sample and method of contact?

Step 6: Specify the group of subjects to be studied

In this step, the researcher must decide specifically who is to be included in the study. The individuals to be studied are known as **research subjects**, while the **population** refers to all the elements – that is, individuals, objects, events or substances – that meet the criteria for inclusion in a given (identified) universe. The definition of the population will depend on the sample criteria and the similarity of subjects in these various settings. The researcher must determine which population is accessible and can be best represented by the study sample. It is usually impossible for the researcher to study all subjects in a population – instead, he/she must use a sample of that population. The researcher will have to finalise the criteria that are to be used in the selection of the sample, as well as decide how to ensure the representativeness of the sample, what sampling method to use and what size the sample should be.

Phase 2: The empirical phase

In this phase, the researcher implements all the plans that he/she made in Phase 1 to collect the data. In many studies, the empirical phase is the most time-consuming part of the investigation. The amount of time spent, however, varies from study to study.

Step 7: Conduct a pilot study of the research

Until this point, only conceptual decision-making and planning has taken place. Now, the researcher is ready to implement the plan. However, where possible, he/she should first carry out a pilot study, which is a small-scale version or 'dummy run' of the major study. Unforeseen problems can arise in the course of a project. By doing a pilot study, the researcher can recognise and address some of the problems by obtaining information for improving the project, making adjustments to the instrument, or re-assessing the feasibility of the study.

The pilot study is sometimes viewed as part of the planning phase as it may bring about changes before the actual data collection commences.

Step 8: Collect the data

The researcher normally collects the data according to the pre-established plan. If the study subjects have not been selected from the target population, this needs to be done at this point. Next, the researcher contacts the subjects and any agencies involved to explain the study and to obtain their written, informed consent. The researcher collects the actual information, that is, data, using the instrument that has been developed and tested in the pilot study.

The data collection method will vary according to the design. The researcher may observe, question or measure the most frequently used methods, and may use instruments such as observations, interviews, questionnaires or scales. Worthwhile research demands that each piece of data collected has a purpose that is related to the study's goal and is not collected as 'nice to know' data.

Phase 3: The interpretive phase

The data collected in the empirical phase are not reported in 'raw' form. The researcher must summarise them and subject them to various types of analysis and interpretation.

Step 9: Analyse the data

Before starting to analyse or process the data, the researcher must examine them for completeness and accuracy. Incomplete and inaccurately completed questionnaires can be discarded. Then the researcher must organise the data in an orderly, coherent fashion so that he/she can discern patterns and relationships.

The process of data analysis is determined by the research approach; the researcher will analyse quantitative and qualitative data differently. Furthermore, a descriptive design, an experiment and a grounded theory study will produce different types and amounts of data.

Analysis techniques conducted in quantitative research include descriptive and inferential statistics and sophisticated advanced analysis. These processes are primarily performed by computer. Most researchers will work closely with statistical consultants in analysing quantitative data. Qualitative analysis involves the integration and synthesis of narrative non-numeric data that are reduced to themes and categories with the aid of a coding procedure.

Step 10: Interpret the results

In order to be meaningful, the results obtained from data analysis require interpretation. Interpretation refers to the researcher's act of drawing conclusions and making sense of the results. As part of the process, he/she asks him-/herself these questions:

- What do the results imply?
- What did we actually learn from the data?
- What do the findings mean for others? What is the value of the study for them?
- Should the study encourage change in some of their policies, their curriculum or their assumptions?
- What recommendations can we make for further research?

Phase 4: The communication phase

In the previous phase, the researcher answers the questions he/she posed in the first phase. The job is not completed, however, until the researcher communicates the results of the study to others who may find it useful.

Step 11: Communicate the research findings

Without a scientific research report, the research process is incomplete. Communication of findings involves the development and dissemination of a research report to appropriate audiences. The report must communicate each step of the study process, and indicates the final product. It should be well organised, informative and succinct.

The researcher should be familiar with the correct way to write a report as well as the publication policies of the various research journals. In the report, the researcher conveys the knowledge and findings of the study in a scientific and intelligible way. The report must also be accurate, objective, clear, concise, consistent and relevant. Furthermore, the researcher's writing style should be appropriate for the readers, be they scientists or lay-persons. Finally, the correct technical presentation of a research report contributes to the scientific value of the study and is thus of vital importance.

Summary

In this chapter, we provided an overview of the major phases and steps of the research process. The process was depicted as a model, which, while giving an idealised view of reality, is nevertheless useful as a guide for the performance of research. The model divides the process into phases and steps, which assists the researcher in preparing a flexible schedule for the time to be spent on each phase. While we presented the phases and steps sequentially, we also pointed out and emphasised their interdependent and interrelated nature. In this chapter our model is particularly applicable to quantitative research.

Exercises

Complete these exercises:
1 Read a research article that interests you. Can you identify the steps of the research process? If not, what is missing? Discuss with your colleagues what the significance of the missing step or steps might be.
2 Select and describe a common health problem, then outline the steps that a researcher should take in order to study the problem scientifically.
3 If you were to do a research study on stigmatisation of HIV-positive teenagers, what would the various steps entail?

5 Selecting or identifying research problems

LEARNING OUTCOMES

On completion of this chapter, you should be able to demonstrate your understanding of
- the process of selecting a research topic
- the terms 'research topic', 'research problem' and 'research purpose'
- sources of researchable problems and how to illustrate each source
- the selection of a research topic in relation to researchability, feasibility, expertise, interest and importance in health sciences
- the correct formulation of a research problem.

Introduction

In Chapter 4 we learnt that the first step in the research process is identifying a problem area or finding a topic of interest to research. This is essential in conducting both quantitative and qualitative research. The problem gives direction to the subsequent steps of the research process. The problem is also the primary focus in a research report. It is therefore important that the producer – that is, the researcher – and the consumer – that is, the reader – of research have a working knowledge of the process of identifying and selecting a research topic.

What is a research topic?

A research topic is a broad problem area that contains numerous potential research problems. Also referred to as a 'concept', the 'phenomenon of interest to the researcher', or the 'domain of enquiry', it acts as the basis for the generating of questions. The topic focuses on areas pertaining to the health sciences, and can be categorised in several major areas, each with an abundance of topics:
- Health sciences practice.
- Health sciences education.
- Health sciences management.
- History or ethics in health sciences.
- Person- or situation-based variables.

Before identifying the research problem, the researcher needs to pose the following important questions:
- Am I sufficiently interested in the topic to maintain my interest and involvement throughout?
- Is the topic researchable in terms of time, resources and availability or accessibility of data?
- Is the topic of value or interest to health care professionals or the broader population? Is there a need for such research?
- Can the results contribute to the body of knowledge for the health sciences?
- Do I want to present the topic in the form of a dissertation or thesis, or publish it as an article in a scholarly journal?

Although choosing a research topic is often difficult, the researcher needs to be patient and considerate so as to minimise the occurrence of problems later in the research process.

Research problem and purpose

The word 'problem', like the word 'science', has several meanings. Whatever the meaning, the problem itself should be clearly formulated. Burns and Grove (2003) describe the **research problem** as an area of concern in which there is a gap or a situation in need of solution, improvement or alteration, or in which there is a discrepancy between the ways things are and the way they ought to be. These problematic situations or discrepancies stimulate interest and prompt investigation. A researcher can identify a problem by asking questions such as the following:

- What is wrong, or of concern, in this situation?
- What is the significance of this problem?
- What is the gap in the knowledge of the situation?
- Will a particular intervention work in a clinical situation?
- What changes need to be made to improve this situation?

It is also possible that a research problem is formulated from sources other than a problematic situation, such as a specific interest in a certain topic. For example, a critical analysis of music therapy for unborn babies, or the use of the radio as media for health education in rural communities. In some instances, existing research is replicated to extend the depth of research in a particular field. Furthermore, topics of social relevance and their practical implications, such as new health-related legislation, need to be investigated.

The **research purpose** is generated from the problem. It clearly and concisely states the aim of the study, for example to explore, describe, identify or predict a solution to the problem. Therefore, the research purpose captures the essence of the study in a single sentence, including the variables, the population and often also the research setting.

Origins of research problems

Research problems are developed from many sources, such as clinical practice; literature; theory; ethical dilemmas; observed health and illness patterns; interaction with colleagues, students, individuals and communities; and established research priorities. Researchers often use more than one of these sources. The sources we describe in this book are clinical practice, literature and theory.

Table 5.1 on the next page illustrates how each of these areas can influence the generation of ideas for a research problem.

The sources we discuss in Table 5.1 serve as examples of common sources; they are by no means inclusive of all possible sources. Whenever you find yourself surprised, frustrated or puzzled, or whenever you express a complaint, a wish, a question or a hope, this is the basis for a research problem.

Table 5.1 The influence of selected sources on the development of a research idea

Source	Influence	Example
A Clinical practice	The health care professional may identify problem areas: ■ through observations ■ in patient assessment interactions ■ in interaction with others ■ in the application or implementation of treatment	■ A health care professional working in a medical ward may observe that patients do not comply with their treatment programmes once they are discharged, despite patient education programmes. He/she therefore recognises that *patient compliance* is a problem area which requires more attention ■ A health care professional working in a clinic in a specific community may observe a much higher proportion of obese teenagers than he/she has saw in other areas. He/she may then identify obesity as a problem area ■ A health care professional working in a surgical ward may observe a difference in the length of time needed for wounds to heal on patients with similar wounds but receiving different dressings. He/she therefore recognises wound dressings as the problem area
B Health sciences literature	The health care professional may find contradictory information or gaps in literature The health care professional may also identify studies to replicate	A health care professional working in a surgical ward reads two research articles on methods to promote pain relief in intravenous infiltration. One writer recommends that warmth should be applied to the infusion site when there is infiltration, while the other recommends cold applications. The question is: Which of the two methods is the most reliable as far as pain and induration relief is concerned? The problem areas in this case would be methods to promote pain relief in intravenous infiltration
C Theory	Theories such as Orem's self-care theory, people's interaction theory, stress theory, motivation theory and so on, may form the basis for research. The health sciences researcher could ask: If this theory is correct, what are the implications for people's behaviours, states or feelings in certain situations?	A health care professional could decide to explore or describe a concept in a theory such as the concept of self-care in Orem's theory or he/she could decide to investigate the success of self-management of a particular condition such as hypertension. Another health care professional may select a learning principle from Roger's theory to test in a patient education programme

Considerations regarding research problems

The researcher needs to consider the following factors when trying to decide if a problem is appropriate for a research study:

- The significance of the study for the health sciences.
- The researchability of the problem.
- The feasibility of the study.
- The ethical acceptability of the study.

Significance to the health sciences

The research study should have the potential to contribute to health sciences knowledge in a meaningful way. If other researchers and scientists commonly react to the study results by asking: 'So what?', the study may well be insignificant or useless. In order to avoid this situation, the researcher should ask these questions:

- Is the problem important for the health sciences?
- Is the research worth doing? If so, why?
- Will patients, health care professionals or the broader community benefit from the findings of this study?
- Will the body of health sciences knowledge be increased as a result of this study?
- Could the findings help to improve health care practice or policies?
- Would implementation of the findings be cost-effective?

If the answer to all these questions is 'yes', the problem has significance for the health sciences. If the answer is 'no' to any of these questions, the researcher should either revise or discard the problem.

Researchability of the problem

Not all questions are amenable to scientific investigation. Research cannot answer a question that is a matter of opinion or philosophy. Value-orientated or 'should' questions may require philosophical analysis and study, rather than research. Examples of such questions are as follows:

- Should heart transplants be performed in provincial hospitals?
- Should all abortions on demand be allowed?
- Should additional clinical experience be included in the psychology curriculum?
- What should the home-based caregiver's role be in the HIV/Aids pandemic?

These questions involve values and opinions, and are therefore not truly researchable. However, they can be *revised* to focus on the beliefs and perceptions of the subjects, or on the impact of the proposed action, and the problem may then be researchable. For example, the first of the preceding questions could be restated as follows: 'How favourably does the community view the moratorium on heart transplants?'.

It is also impossible to research the type of question that can be answered by a simple 'yes' or 'no'. For example:

- Do most lecturers in South Africa have a Masters degree?
- Are patients in Ward X kept waiting for pain medication after they request it?

Data could be collected to answer the question posed, but the problems do not relate to a broader theoretical problem to offer explanations or make predictions. To qualify as 'researchable', the questions must be transformed so as to suggest a reason for the researcher collecting the information needed to answer them. For example, the second of the preceding questions may be restated as: 'What are the consequences of keeping patients waiting for pain medication after they request it?'.

A researchable question is one that yields facts to solve a problem, generate new research, add to theory or improve health care practice. A question that will elicit answers that explain, describe, identify, substantiate, predict or qualify is a researchable question (Brink & Wood 1994; Burns & Grove 2003).

Feasibility of the study

Many potentially interesting and researchable questions have to be discarded because they are not feasible. To assess the feasibility of a study, the researcher must answer a number of questions, such as the following:

- Can this research be done in the time that is available?
- Will available resources – that is, money, equipment and facilities – be sufficient to complete the study?
- Can a sufficient number of research subjects be located and, if so, will they be willing to cooperate?
- Are there appropriate instruments or techniques available to study the problem?
- Will I be able to get approval from the relevant authorities to undertake this project?
- Do I have the expertise to undertake this study?
- Am I sufficiently interested in the study?

Time availability

The first-time researcher is likely to have difficulty in trying to assess how much work is involved, and how long it will take. A good starting point for attempting the assessment is for the researcher to use, as a framework, the various steps of the research process that we discuss in Chapter 4. Each step in the process can be broken down into as much detail as possible, and time can be allocated to every step as appropriate. A novice researcher should ask for advice from more experienced researchers. Valuable information about how long literature searches will take, and in particular how long it will take to locate and access literature, can also be obtained from librarians.

If ethics committee approval or permission from authorities is required, a study may be delayed for a considerable period of time. The researcher needs to take this into consideration.

Even well-planned research may take longer than expected or planned. The total length of time required should be calculated and an appropriate decision taken as to how much time is necessary for the study. For example, if you are required to do a small research project for an Honours study within six months, and the time you have calculated for your study is one year, your study will not be feasible. You will have to redefine it to 'fit' the time available. Moreover, if you plan or expect to complete a study in one year and the data collection takes longer due to a delay in the return of questionnaire responses, you need to adapt the research plan.

Resources availability

The resource requirements can vary considerably from study to study. Undertaken as part of an Honours course, a study may need nominal resources only, while a much larger project may require vast quantities of both material, such as copies of instruments, and equipment, such as computers, telephones, and so on. The design of the study will also influence the amount of resources required. Costs of processes such as literature searches, photocopying, telephone communication, statistical consultations, typing and report production, as well as of items such as postage, computer access, specialised equipment, travel and office space rental must all be considered. The more detailed the list, the more accurately the feasibility of the study can be assessed. The researcher needs to ask him-/herself: 'Do I or will I have the financial resources required, and does the anticipated cost outweigh the value of the expected finding?'.

Subject availability

In any study involving human subjects, the researcher needs to consider whether enough people with the desired characteristics will be available. Furthermore, it is important to recognise that potential subjects may not be as enthusiastic about the research study as the researcher. Some may refuse to participate, others may be reluctant to complete any questionnaire, and others still may drop out after having initially agreed to participate. The types and numbers of subjects available and their cooperation are key factors in the researcher's determination of whether and how a study can be conducted.

Researcher expertise

It is important that the researcher closely examines the level of expertise required to undertake and successfully complete the identified study. Novice researchers or appraisers of research need to have knowledge of the concepts relevant to conducting research and of the area under study. They must also have the ability to judge the data from various perspectives. They need to take stock of what they know. For example, a health worker wants to do research on health care managers and their leadership strategies, and her stock of information is based entirely on her experience as a health worker. Her study would be useless, because she simply does not know enough. By contrast, she *does* have knowledge of how a health worker is subjected to various management strategies. If she talks to other health workers about their managers, and reads about supervision and management and how it is best accomplished, she may be well on the way to doing research on health workers' perceptions of various managerial and administrative strategies.

Researcher motivation and interest

Motivation is perhaps the most significant prerequisite for undertaking health sciences research and seeing it through. Motivation and enthusiasm are indicative of a person's positive disposition and ability to persist with a task. Successful investigations are dependent upon just such a disposition; an uninterested, passive attitude towards work normally leads to failure. Even if it entails a relatively simple project, research takes time, and requires considerable thought and organisation. It is therefore of the utmost importance that researchers are genuinely interested in the topic or project they select for research.

The research problem does not exist in a vacuum

The identified problem area does not exist in a vacuum – it is embedded in a particular context. Moreover, the researcher will view the problem from a particular perspective, which itself will depend on the researcher's philosophical position. This means that the researcher will have a set of beliefs, values and assumptions which will influence the way he/she perceives human beings, the environment, health and health care.

In addition, the researcher has theoretical and methodological beliefs about the nature and structure of the problem area. The theoretical beliefs are derived from theories, and must be expressed as testable statements also known as 'assumptions'. Methodological beliefs are preferences, assumptions and presuppositions about what ought to constitute good research. Any decisions made by the researcher with regard to the pursuit of the problem will be guided by these beliefs, which will also define the boundaries and directions of the project, as we discussed in Chapter 2.

Ethical acceptability of the study

In health sciences research, human beings are usually the subjects of the study. The researcher has the responsibility of considering whether the study at hand will be ethical. Research should never be done at the expense of human beings, a point which we explored in detail in Chapter 3. Professional ethics are increasingly being taken into account by researchers in the planning and conducting of their research.

Formulation of a research problem

When formulating a research problem, the researcher should follow these guidelines:

- Formulate the research problem as an open-ended question. For example: What are the educational requirements for self-management of hypertension?
- Alternatively, formulate a statement. For example: Educational guidelines have an effect on the self-management of hypertension.
- Include the research design to be used. For example: The development of a short course in trauma counselling: A case study of Sunshine Hospice. In this example a *case study* would be done to address the research problem.
- Include the actions or interventions to solve the research problem. For example: The development of a model for support of caregivers of Aids orphans and vulnerable children. In this example the *development of a model* is the action that would address the research problem.

Summary

In this chapter, we focused on the process of identifying and selecting a research topic and problem. We defined the terms 'research topic', 'research problem' and 'research purpose'. As well as giving examples of sources of research studies, we explored the factors that the researcher must consider when selecting a research problem. We concluded the chapter with a set of guidelines for the formulation of a research problem.

Exercises

Complete these exercises:

1 Discuss at least five sources which could provide research problems for study in the health sciences.
2 In what circumstances would a problem be inappropriate for scientific research?
3 Distinguish between a research problem and a research purpose.

6 The literature review

LEARNING OUTCOMES

On completion of this chapter, you should be able to demonstrate your understanding of

- the reasons for a literature review being an essential part of every project
- the purpose of a literature review
- the differences between primary and secondary sources
- the steps of the review process
- how to locate appropriate references for the research topic
- the guidelines for writing a literature review
- a framework for evaluating a literature review.

Introduction

Once the researcher has identified the topic and the purpose of the study, he/she must conduct a systematic *search of the literature* to find out precisely what is known about the topic. The 'literature' refers to the sources that are effective in providing the in-depth knowledge that the researcher needs to study the selected problem.

The literature search and review is a crucial element of the research process – it frequently means the difference between a focused, thorough and well-designed study and one that is fragmented, incomplete and poorly planned. A thorough examination of publications on the topic is essential to developing an understanding of a given area, to limiting the scope of the study and to conveying the importance of studying the topic. Overlooking the literature can lead to the ineffective development of a research project that will not serve to improve health care or health sciences practice.

According to Burns and Grove (2005: 93),

> a literature review is an organized written presentation of what has been published on a topic by scholars. The purpose of the review is to convey to the reader what is currently known regarding the topic of interest.

In most studies a literature review is done at the onset of the study and is updated or extended during the final phase. The review helps the researcher to decide whether the topic can and should be researched.

As a result of the sudden and huge increase of knowledge and the accessibility of computerised databases, reviewing the literature has become an exciting and stimulating experience, though the risk of plagiarism has been concomitantly heightened.

Definitions

The literature is all the written sources relevant to the topic of interest. A literature review involves finding, reading, understanding and forming conclusions about the published research and theory as well as presenting it in an organised manner (Burns & Grove 2005).

Purpose of the literature review

The researcher conducts the literature review for various reasons:

- To conduct a critical analytical appraisal of the recent scholarly work on the topic. By determining what is already known about the topic, the researcher can obtain a comprehensive picture of the state of knowledge.
- To identify the research problem and refine the research questions.

■ To place the study in the context of the general body of knowledge, which minimises the possibility of unintentional duplication and increases the probability that the new study makes a valuable contribution.

■ To obtain clues to the methodology and instruments. This aspect provides the researcher with information on what has and has not been attempted with regard to approaches and methods, and on what types of data-collecting instruments exist and work or do not work.

■ To refine certain parts of the study, specifically the problem statement, hypothesis, conceptual framework, design and data analysis process.

■ To compare the findings of existing studies with those of the study at hand. This process shows the relevance of the latter findings to the existing body of knowledge.

■ To inform or support a qualitative study, especially in conjunction with the collection and analysis of data.

The specific aims of the literature review depend on the role of the researcher. He/she can use the review to acquire knowledge on the topic or to critique existing practices; to develop research-based protocols and interventions; to develop a theory or conceptual framework; or to develop policy statements, curricula or practice guidelines (Polit, Beck & Hungler 2001).

Types of information and sources

Polit, Beck and Hungler (2001) divide the types of information to be included in a literature review into the following five categories:
1 Facts, statistics and research findings.
2 Theories or interpretations.
3 Methods and procedures.
4 Opinions, beliefs or points of view.
5 Anecdotes, clinical impressions or narrations of incidents and situations.

Facts, statistics and research findings

This category constitutes one of the most important types of information for a literature review. Research findings can suggest topics for investigation, and can help the researcher in conceptualising and designing new research. Depending on the topic, it is usually useful for the researcher to review research findings in the health sciences literature as well as in the literature of related disciplines, such as sociology, psychology, anthropology, education and management. A good literature review should include current literature as well as material of historical interest.

Theories or interpretations

This category deals with broader, more conceptual issues of relevance. For example, if you wish to research stress in students, you would search the literature for various stress theories; if you are concerned with the particular needs of certain patients, you would search for theories on patient needs. Descriptions of theories are useful in providing a conceptual context for a research problem.

Methods and procedures

In this category, the researcher deals with information concerning the methods of conducting a study; that is, in reviewing the literature, the researcher should pay attention not only to *what* has been found but also to *how* it was found. He/she needs to pose these questions:

- What approaches have other researchers used?
- How have they operationalised and measured their variables?
- How have they controlled the research situation to enhance interpretation?
- What statistical methods have they used to analyse the data?

Opinions, beliefs or points of view

Articles focusing on authors' opinions or attitudes are inherently subjective, and present the suggestions and points of view of one or several individuals. If the study focuses on controversial or emerging issues in the health care sciences, 'opinion articles' may be a valuable source of ideas.

Anecdotes, clinical impressions or narrations of incidents and situations

This category may serve to broaden the researcher's understanding of the problem, particularly if he/she is relatively unfamiliar with the underlying issues. Such sources may also illustrate a point or demonstrate a need for rigorous research. However, the elements in this category have limited utility in literature reviews for research studies because of their highly subjective nature. The researcher should not rely heavily on such sources in his/her review of the literature.

Primary and secondary sources

Primary sources are those in which the data are reported and written by the person or group that actually gathered the information, or conducted the investigation. There are two broad types of primary data sources – research studies and statistical reports. While the latter is self-explanatory, **research studies** range in scope from the small pilot study to broad-based, controlled experiments. In the health care sciences, primary sources of information also include diaries, letters, interviews, eyewitness accounts, speeches, documents and autobiographies.

Secondary sources are those in which the reporter of the information is not the person or group that actually obtained the data; therefore, the information can be regarded as second-hand. Secondary sources summarise or quote content from primary sources, which means that authors of secondary sources paraphrase the work of researchers and theorists. The problem with this is that the author has interpreted the work of someone else, and that the interpretation is influenced by the author's perceptions and bias. As a result, errors and misinterpretations have been promulgated by authors using secondary rather than primary sources. The researcher should strive to locate and utilise primary material when undertaking a study, because it provides the least biased raw material.

Format of the available literature

Common formats used to convey information include
- journals
- books
- reports
- theses and dissertations
- conference proceedings
- government circulars
- computer databases.

Clearly, the researcher has a wide variety of formats from which to choose.

Depth and breadth of the review

The **depth** of a literature review refers to the number and quality of the sources that the researcher examines. The **breadth** is determined by the number of different sources examined. If the literature review is too broad, the researcher will examine many irrelevant sources. When the review lacks sufficient depth and breadth, the researcher may overlook important sources. The depth and breadth of the literature review depend on the background of the researcher, the complexity of the research topic, and the amount of relevant literature that is available. The literature review should be broad enough for the researcher to be knowledgeable about the research problem and narrow enough to include predominantly relevant sources.

The review process

In the process of reviewing the literature in quantitative and qualitative research, the researcher should
- use the library
- identify sources

- locate sources
- critically read sources
- write the review report
- evaluate the review report.

Use the library

Irrespective of the topic of interest, it is highly unlikely that the researcher will have all the required literature at hand. For most researchers it is necessary to use a library as the main source of their research literature. Not all libraries are the same; some offer more services than others. The researcher who intends to use a particular library must acquaint him-/herself with its facilities and staff. The librarian can assist him/her in the use of the card catalogue, the various indexes and other reference materials, as well as with computer-assisted searches. Moreover, the librarian can inform the researcher about the administration of the library with regard to working hours, photocopy services, check-out policies and interlibrary loan materials.

Identify sources

In conducting an in-depth search of the literature, the researcher must first clarify the research topic and then identify all relevant publications in the area of interest. 'Relevance' refers to how closely the information relates to the topic. For example, a researcher who is interested in studying the relationship between obesity and dietary patterns in teenagers would try to find

- research that examines the same question
- research that examines related questions, for example the eating patterns of successful dieters, factors influencing obesity, diets in obesity, the general eating patterns of teenagers
- information relating to the concepts of obesity, teenagers and dietary patterns
- information relating to the characteristics of obese teenagers.

There are several basic **types of resources** for the search:

- The database of books and journals available in the library system. Generally, the catalogue contains an alphabetical listing of books in three categories, according to title, author and subject heading. Today these are available electronically.
- The indexes covering various fields of study. Indexes are frequently used to find journal or periodical references. Examples of such indexes are the International Nursing Index (INI), the Cumulative Index to Nursing and Allied Health Literature (CINAHL) and Index Medicus.
- The indexes printed at the end of each year for most journals.
- Abstracts. These comprise brief summaries of articles. The Dissertation Abstracts International is a comprehensive source for doctoral dissertations.

■ Computer-assisted literature searches. There are many computer databases, the following being some of the most useful to researchers:
  ❑ Nursing and Allied Health. The CINAHL CD-ROM provides access to this database.
  ❑ Medline. This database corresponds to three printed indexes, namely, Index Medicus, INI and the Index to Dental Literature. Access to this database is online and via CD-ROM.
■ Local resources. These may not be found in all libraries, but some that can be consulted at the relevant institutions are
  ❑ the completed research lists of the Human Sciences Research Council (HSRC), the Medical Research Council (MRC), the National Research Foundation (NRF) and professional bodies
  ❑ the joint catalogue of theses and dissertations of South African universities.

In computer searches, keywords and phrases are entered into a computer program and a list of relevant articles can be obtained and printed out. Novice researchers will need the assistance of a librarian, or some other experienced person, when using this resource. Health care professionals working in isolated rural areas and in smaller centres may not have access to these facilities. We suggest that they talk to people who know something about the topic, and that they also look through the most recent journals for pertinent articles. The list of references at the end of the articles usually provide information on further appropriate literature, and in this way the researchers can build up a substantial literature list.

Locate sources

In order to locate the sources, the researcher must follow these steps:
■ Organise the list of identified sources.
■ Search the library for those sources.
■ Systematically record the references.
■ Determine additional ways to locate sources.

Organise the list of identified sources, and search the library for them

The researcher can organise the list in several ways to facilitate locating them in the library. Journal sources could be organised by journal name and year of publication. For example, if most of the articles on the list are from the *Journal of Advanced Nursing, Nursing Research*, the *Journal of Nursing Education* and the *International Nursing Review*, the researcher would group the articles from each of these journals together and organise them according to the year of publication. This prevents the researcher from simply wandering from one journal to the next.

The researcher can facilitate his/her search for sources in the library by talking to library personnel and familiarising him-/herself with the layout and organisation of the library. He/she can save time by finding out where books, journals, reports and dictionaries are located, and how they are classified. Larger reports, articles and shorter reports usually have to be scanned and summarised immediately, as students are seldom allowed to take these documents out of the library. A memory stick is valuable for downloading some of the electronic articles or other sources to read at a later stage. Researchers must familiarise themselves with the copyright policies of their institutions.

Systematically record the references

It is necessary that the researcher establishes a systematic method for recording pertinent information. While there are many such methods, it is often suggested that each article be entered separately by hand on a card. For ease of use, the cards can be kept in alphabetical order by author or title. Researchers who have access to a computer can enter the same information rather than using cards. Each entry should include the

- author(s) name(s)
- date of publication
- title of the article, report or book
- name of the journal or publisher
- volume and number of the journal
- place of publication, if it is a book
- page numbers on which the material appears
- initial notes you have made about it.

The notes that the researcher makes on the articles should contain the

- problem statement
- definition of concepts
- hypotheses, if any
- theories or assumptions used
- method of research, if applicable
- instruments used, if applicable
- data analysis, if applicable
- findings and summaries
- researcher's evaluation of each aspect.

Careful note-taking and reference citation are extremely useful, and facilitate the rest of the research process. A systematic recording process also increases the accuracy of the references in the researcher's research report. Computer software packages such as EndNote and Reference Manager can be used to organise references.

Determine additional ways to locate sources

Even the largest libraries do not contain *every* text for which the researcher may have a relevant reference. The researcher may need to use the interlibrary loan service, which is done with the assistance of the librarian. Note that the process, which entails locating and accessing a text from another library, can be time consuming.

Critically read sources

Critical reading involves a preliminary phase and a critical review. In the **preliminary phase** the researcher reads the abstract and scans the article, chapter or report in order to determine whether it is suitable for the purpose of the review. Then he/she **critically reviews** the relevant pieces. This entails analysing the usability, completeness and consistency of the piece, evaluating its strengths and weaknesses, and assessing its relationship with the study at hand. The critical review helps the researcher to evaluate every decision taken in each step of the research process.

Write the review report

When writing the literature review, the researcher reviews the literature in some detail, but as a rule does not report on the whole of the literature review. It is not appropriate for the researcher to try to include everything, and he/she should rather report on the portions of the review which are presumed to be relevant, that is, directly related to the problem and purpose of the proposed study. Nevertheless, it is essential that the reported review is scientifically adequate, or clinically applicable.

The researcher must pay particular attention to the following:

- The literature review should represent a thoughtful analysis and synthesis of the literature, and not just a collection of quotations and conclusions. Gathering together quotes from various documents fails to show whether the existing research and thought on the topic have been assimilated and understood.
- The literature review should start with an introduction. The introduction should refer to the sources consulted, and give an indication of the amount of work that is in existence. In addition, the introduction should briefly describe the structure and purpose of the review, so as to guide the reader and contextualise all the elements.
- The main body of the review should consist of the critique of existing work, as well as the theoretical dimension. The researcher should begin by describing the scholarly literature on the independent variable, and should then discuss the dependent variable(s) and their relationships.
- The content of the sources should be paraphrased or summarised in the researcher's own words, and should reveal the current state of knowledge on the selected subject.
- Direct quotes may be used to emphasise central issues. If used, they should be kept as short as possible. Long quotes are often unnecessary, and tend to interfere

with the reader's train of thought. Moreover, quotes should be reproduced identically, and care should be taken that they are not used out of context as the significance may be lost, or the reader may misinterpret them.

- Full credit must be given to authors for all statements taken from their work, be it directly or indirectly. If this is not done, the researcher is guilty of plagiarism, and is liable for prosecution. Due credit is given to the authors by indicating their name(s) and the year of publication between parentheses immediately following the statement. Moreover, full details of author(s), publication date, title, publisher and place of publication must be provided in a reference list at the end of the chapter or text. There are different systems according to which the list of references may be exactly compiled, for example the Harvard system, the adapted Harvard system and the Vancouver system. One of these is not necessarily more correct than another, but whichever system is used, it must be applied consistently.
- The review should be as objective as possible. A text that fails to support the researcher's hypothesis or that conflicts with his/her personal values should not be omitted. Material which has been obtained from sources should be presented honestly, and not be distorted to support the selected problem.
- The review should be balanced, identifying the strengths and weaknesses of each of the references, and should compare differences and similarities among them. In other words, the review must reflect all sides of the issue.
- The review should include the most up-to-date information.
- The review should conclude with a summary of the synthesised findings of the existing work, which should clearly describe the extent of the current knowledge base. The summary should also point out gaps in the literature, or areas of 'research inactivity'.

Evaluate the research review

Researchers have to evaluate not only the literature that they review, but also their own written review. Some relevant questions that need to be posed in this process are as follows:

- Is the review comprehensive?
- Is it relevant to the problem at hand?
- Is it up to date?
- Are all sides of the issue presented?
- Is there enough sound research-based evidence?
- Is the use of secondary sources excessive?
- Does it critically appraise the contribution of key studies?
- Is it logically organised?
- Does it attempt to be sufficiently objective?

Summary

In this chapter, we explained that the main functions of a literature review are to provide an up-to-date account of what is known about the study topic, to provide a conceptual and theoretical context, to assist the researcher in obtaining clues to the methodology and instrumentation, and to refine certain parts of the study. We pointed out that the type of information to be included in the review is divided into five broad categories, and that literature sources are classified as either primary or secondary. We discussed in detail the five steps or components of the review process, in which we proposed that the review should present a thoughtful analysis of the field, and not simply a collection of quotations and summaries. Furthermore, it should include all published points of view, rather than simply those that support the researcher's view. Finally, we pointed out that the literature review must be submitted to the same critical analysis and ethical assessment as the rest of the research process.

Exercises

Complete these exercises:

1 Select a research article from a health sciences journal and evaluate its literature review according to the guidelines set out in this chapter. We suggest the following articles for reinforcing our points:

Kemp, MG, Keithley, JK, Smith, DW and Morreale, B. 1990. Factors that contribute to pressure sores in surgical patients. *Research in Nursing and Health* 13, 293–301.

Maloni, JA, Chance, B, Zhang, C, Cohen, AW, Betts, D and Gange, S. 1993. Physical and psychosocial side effects of antepartum hospital bedrest: A review of the literature. *Image* 233, 187–97.

2 Comment on the following aspects in the research article that you selected in the first exercise:

   a) The relevance of the literature to the problem area.
   b) The use of primary sources and secondary sources.
   c) The current nature of the literature.
   d) The use of empirical material versus theory and opinion.

3 Imagine that you want to research the post-operative experiences of female patients. List the key concepts and phrases which you think would aid your literature search.

4 Visit your academic library and locate the card catalogue, indexes and abstracts in texts about the health sciences, and discuss how to arrange interlibrary loans. Perform an electronic database search, and even try the Cochrane Library.

7 Refining and defining the research question or formulating a hypothesis and preparing a research proposal

LEARNING OUTCOMES

On completion of this chapter, you should be able to demonstrate your understanding of

■ the purpose, objectives, questions and hypotheses of research projects

■ the essential aspects in formulating a research question, objective and hypothesis

■ the different types of hypotheses

■ the different variables

■ conceptual and operational definitions

■ the types of studies for which hypotheses are not needed

■ the significance and preparation of a research proposal.

Introduction

The researcher must transform the general topic into a manageable, researchable problem that indicates exactly what is going to be studied. This transformation takes time and requires creative thinking. One way of conducting the process is through asking a series of questions linked to the area of concern, and then defining specific factors that might be studied. During this process the researcher also considers the suitability of the quantitative or the qualitative research approaches. The selection of the research approach is finalised once the research topic and problem have been clarified.

Refining the researchable problem

Refining the research problem entails the conscious exercise of choice in order to formalise the identified problem or area of interest. For example, a researcher works in a clinic and has identified his/her area of concern to be obesity in teenagers. Questions that may arise are as follows:

- What dietary patterns do these teenagers follow?
- If a weight reduction protocol is prescribed, will they comply? If so, will this lead to successful weight loss?

Several potential research problems could result from this exercise, such as the following:

- What dietary patterns do obese teenagers follow?
- Is there a relationship between compliance with a weight reduction protocol and successful weight loss in obese teenagers?
- How effective is a weight reduction protocol on the incidence of weight loss in obese teenagers?
- How do obese teenagers experience their obesity?

These problems have a similar theme, yet each one is unique and can be studied in a different manner. Each has a specific focus, is clearly worded and can give direction to the study. Each has thus been transformed into a manageable, researchable problem.

These problems are formulated as questions. The researcher can now establish the purpose for conducting the study. The purpose statement should include

- the aim of the research, specified with terms such as 'to identify', 'to describe', 'to explore', 'to explain' and 'to predict'
- the target population
- the setting
- the research variables.

For example: 'The purpose of this study is to describe the dietary patterns of obese teenagers in community X'. In this example, the aim is to describe, the target population is obese teenagers, the setting is community X and the research variable is dietary patterns. In this case only a single variable is described. If the purpose of the study, for example, is to determine the efficacy of a weight reduction protocol on the incidence of weight loss in obese teenagers residing in community X, two variables would have to be considered, namely, weight reduction protocol and weight loss.

Having formulated the research problem and purpose, the researcher needs to pose the following questions to determine whether the area of concern has been properly addressed:

- Does the problem statement address the area of concern clearly and concisely?
- Is the purpose clearly formulated?
- Will it be feasible to study the problem and purpose?
- Does the purpose clarify or limit the focus or aim of the study?
- Will the problem and purpose generate knowledge for the field of interest?
- Will the purpose of the study be ethical?
- Am I sufficiently experienced to conduct the study?
- Will the findings of the study have an impact on health care?

Research objectives, questions or hypotheses grow out of the more abstractly stated research problem and purpose, once these have been examined for significance and feasibility. The objectives are formulated to bridge the gap between the problem and purpose and the detailed design and plan for data collection and analysis. Most writers differentiate only between questions and hypotheses. However, Burns and Grove (2003), whose example we are following, differentiate between objectives, questions and hypotheses.

Research objectives

An 'objective' is a concrete, measurable end towards which effort or ambition is directed. Research objectives are therefore defined as clear, concise, declarative statements that are written in the present tense. An objective usually focuses on one or two variables, and indicates whether the variables are to be identified, analysed or described. At times, the focus of an objective includes identifying relationships among variables and determining differences between two groups regarding selected variables.

Researchers may state objectives in cases where minimal or no research on a problem exists, and when the purpose of the study is to identify or describe characteristics of variables or to identify relationships among variables. A study done, for example, on the magnitude of lower back problems in health care professionals demonstrates the logical flow from research problem and purpose to conducting the research.

Example 1

The purpose of the study is to describe the magnitude of lower back problems in health care professionals.

The objectives of the study are to
- determine the prevalence of lower back problems in health care professionals
- ascertain differences between health care professionals who had occupational lower back problems and those without lower back problems in relation to age, work experience and perceived amount of lifting of patients per shift
- determine the amount of work time lost, the amount of change in daily activities, the perceived precipitating factors, if any, and the setting in which the lower back problems occur
- determine whether health care professionals have considered leaving the profession because of the lower back problems.

This example clearly illustrates that the objectives flow logically from the research problem and purpose, and that they refine the problem and purpose and provide greater detail on what the researcher is going to research.

Research questions

While a research objective is a *declarative* statement, a research question is an *interrogative* statement. Research questions are used for the same purposes as objectives. In fact, many writers, among them Polit and Hungler (1995) and Breakwell, Hammond and Fife-Schaw (2000), refer to questions *and* objectives as questions, while distinguishing between them according to the form in which they are stated. Babbie and Mouton (2001) regard research questions as being synonymous with research problems, except that they are stated in question form.

Here follows an example of how a research purpose is refined into a research question using the interrogative form. The study is on the portrayal of nurses in advertisements in medical and other health-related journals.

Example 2

The purpose of the study is to examine the content of advertisements in medical and other health-related journals to determine if the images of nurses reflect the roles that the nurses play in health care.

The following questions are addressed in this study:

- What are the images of nurses portrayed in advertisements in medical and other health-related journals?
- Are there differences between the images of nurses and those of physicians when both appear in the same advertisement?
- Do the images of the roles of nurses differ from the actual roles that nurses play in the health care system?
- Is the portrayal of nurses stereotyped with regard to characteristics such as uniforms and physical appearance?

When contrasted with the research purpose, the research questions are more precise. They flow from the research purpose, and they narrow the focus of the study.

Research questions that are formulated for qualitative studies are generally broader in focus and include concepts that are more complex and abstract than in quantitative studies. The following is an example of a qualitative study.

Example 3

The purpose of the study is to explore the characteristics of women who successfully manage their weight.

The following questions are addressed in this study:

- What methods for weight management are used by women who successfully manage their weight?
- What factors influence the selection of the particular methods?

From the above examples we can see that the problem, purpose, objectives and questions need to be clear, logical and focused on the area of concern in the study framework, and moreover that they direct the remaining steps of the research process.

Research hypotheses

A hypothesis is a set of assumptions expressed in a coherent manner about the observable phenomena. It is the formal statement comprising the researcher's prediction or explanation of the relationship between two or more variables in a specific population. In other words, the hypothesis translates the problem statement into a prediction of expected outcomes which is based on theoretical considerations.

Hypotheses are typically used in quantitative research to direct correlational, quasi-experimental or experimental studies, and to test theories. Hypotheses sometimes follow directly from a theoretical framework. The researcher reasons from theories to hypotheses, and tests the hypotheses in the real world. Hypotheses have to be tested empirically before they can be accepted and incorporated into a theory. If a hypothesis is not supported by empirical evidence, it must be rejected and the researcher is obliged to suggest a different hypothesis. In this sense, the role of the hypothesis is not only to make predictions or to explain certain facts or problems but also to guide the investigation and provide a focus for the study.

The following are the main characteristics of usable hypotheses:

- A hypothesis must state the predicted relationship between two or more variables. In the example, 'Persons with Type 2 diabetes who have greater knowledge of their disease will have a higher rate of adherence to the treatment regimen than persons with lesser knowledge', the predicted relationship is between knowledge and adherence to the treatment regimen. Knowledgeable persons will have a higher rate of adherence, while persons with little knowledge will have a low rate. This can be regarded as a workable hypothesis, as it contains two concepts that are likely to vary, namely, adherence and knowledge.

Let us consider whether the following statement relates to workable research: 'Persons with Type 2 diabetes who follow a structured programme on their condition have a high rate of adherence to the treatment regimen'. This statement expresses no anticipated relationship; there is only one variable – the person's adherence to treatment. The hypothesis is therefore not amenable to testing. If a hypothesis lacks a phrase such as 'more than', 'less than', 'different from' or 'related to' it is not amenable to scientific testing because there is no criterion for assessing absolute as opposed to relative outcomes. This type of statement cannot be called a 'hypothesis'.

- A hypothesis must be conceptually clear and specific, and stated as simply as possible. All variables identified must be described with the use of operational definitions.
- A hypothesis should be consistent with an existing body of research findings and with logical reasoning. It must not predict results which are inherently contradictory.
- A hypothesis must be testable with available techniques.
- A hypothesis must relate to a matter which can be clearly defined empirically. Expressions such as 'good', 'bad', 'ought to' and 'should' are not scientific and should not form part of a hypothesis.

Types of hypotheses

Many types of hypotheses are described in the literature and appear in published studies. The type of hypothesis formulated in a study is determined by the purpose of the study. The most basic and most frequently quoted classifications are directional versus non-directional, simple versus complex and null versus research.

A **directional hypothesis** predicts an outcome in a specific direction. For example: 'Diabetic patients who have followed a structured programme on their condition will be more compliant than diabetic patients who have not followed a programme'. In this example, 'more ... than' indicates the direction. Phrases such as 'greater than', 'smaller than', 'more than', 'less than', 'positively' and 'negatively' all indicate direction.

The **non-directional hypothesis** indicates that a difference or correlation exists, but it does not specify the anticipated direction. For example: 'There is a correlation between the number of sources of stress reported by health care professionals in South Africa and the health care professionals' desire to leave employment in the South African health profession'.

The directional hypothesis is the preferred type for a health sciences research study if previous studies in the area have demonstrated contradictory findings.

A **simple hypothesis**, which is sometimes also called 'bivariate', contains only two variables, namely, an independent variable and a dependent variable. The mathematical representation of a simple *associative* hypothesis, in which variables X and Y are related to or associated with one another, is:

The mathematical representation of a simple *causal* hypothesis, in which X is the cause of Y, is:

$$X \longrightarrow Y$$

The following are examples of simple hypotheses:
- There is a relationship between self-concept and suicide.
- CPR training has an effect on the emotional stress of family members of cardiac disease patients.

A **complex hypothesis**, also called 'multivariate', predicts the relationships between three or more variables. There may be two or more independent variables, and one or more dependent variable, or vice versa.

The mathematical expression of a complex *causal* hypothesis with two independent variables XI and X2, and one dependent variable Y, is:

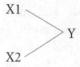

Examples of complex hypotheses are as follows:
- Daily weight loss is greater for adults who follow a reduced calorie diet and exercise daily than for those who do not follow a reduced calorie diet and do not exercise daily.
- Persons who participate in a daily wellness programme have lower stress levels, higher physical functioning and fewer adverse symptoms than those who do not participate in the programme.

The researcher needs to be cautious when using complex hypotheses as these may become difficult to measure within a reasonable time. It may be better to divide a complex hypothesis into simple hypotheses. However, there are times when complex hypotheses are necessary.

The **null hypothesis**, also referred to as 'statistical', is used for statistical testing and for interpreting statistical outcomes. It states that no difference exists between groups; put differently, that there is no correlation between variables. For example: 'There is no relationship between knowledge about HIV and gender'. If there is no statistically significant difference in levels of knowledge of HIV and gender, the null hypothesis is supported, but if a difference in levels of knowledge of HIV between men and women exists, the null hypothesis is rejected.

A **research hypothesis** states that a difference or correlation between two or more variables does exist. All the hypotheses given above are research hypotheses.

Identifying variables

Burns and Grove (2003) define variables as the qualities, properties or characteristics of persons, things or situations that change or vary. Thus, by its nature, a variable can take on more than one possible value. For example, the variable 'gender' can take two values, that is, male and female. The variable 'age' can take many more values, such as below 20 years, 21–30 years, or any number between 0 and 100. The variables 'academic success', 'stress', 'pain' and 'satisfaction' can all take on more than two values at different times.

Types of variables

Since a variable is a quantifiable element that changes or varies, a researcher may have to manage and assess several variables. Some variables can be manipulated; others can be controlled. Some are identified but not measured; others are measured with refined measurement devices.

Independent variables

Also known as a 'treatment' or 'experimental variable', the independent variable influences other variables, thus causing change. It is perceived as contributing to or preceding a particular outcome. In experiments or quasi-experiments, the researcher manipulates the independent variable. The researcher performs intervention or treatment to see the resulting change in the dependent variable.

Dependent variables

The dependent variable is the outcome variable, as it reflects the effect of or response to the independent variable. It is the variable that appears, disappears, diminishes or amplifies – in short, changes – as the experiment introduces, removes or varies the independent variable, for example a study that attempts to demonstrate the effects of an exercise programme in patients with occlusions of some of the major leg arteries. The dependent variables that are measured include the distance walked by the patient to the limit of pain tolerance. The independent variable is the exercise programme, which includes daily walking with the intention of increasing the distance regularly. In another study – to determine the effects of salt intake on hypertension – the blood pressure is the dependent variable, and salt intake is the independent variable.

It is important for you to understand that there is nothing about a variable itself that makes it independent or dependent; the *use* of the variable in the problem under investigation is the crucial factor. For example, in a study to determine the effect of preparation information on post-operative anxiety, anxiety is the dependent variable, while the giving or withholding of preparation information is the independent variable. By contrast, in a study to determine the effects of anxiety on post-surgical pain, anxiety is the independent variable and pain the dependent variable.

Extraneous variables

These are uncontrolled variables that influence the findings of the research study. An extraneous variable impacts on the independent X and dependent Y variables, giving the impression of a relationship between them, when in fact both X and Y change because of the variation of a third variable. In experimental and quasi-experimental research, extraneous variables are of primary concern and are referred to as 'threats' to internal and external validity. Examples are passage of time, mortality, selection bias, instrumentation and maturity.

Extraneous variables are not always recognised, and by their nature they are uncontrolled. Nevertheless, the researcher needs to make the attempt to control them. For these reasons, they may influence the outcomes of the study.

Demographic variables

Also called 'attribute variables', these variables cannot be manipulated or influenced by the researcher, yet they may be present and may vary in the population under study. Examples are characteristics of the research subjects such as gender, age, race, marital status, religion and educational level, which are inherent to the subjects before the study begins.

The researcher analyses these variables to form a picture of the sample.

Research variables

Research variables are measurable concepts in research studies in which a single phenomenon is being examined. They are the logical groupings of attributes, characteristics or traits of the phenomenon. Identified in the research purpose and in the observed objectives or questions, they are used when the researcher intends to observe or measure variables in their natural setting, without implementing a treatment. Therefore, there is neither manipulation of an independent variable nor examination of a cause–effect relationship. For example: A qualitative study to describe patients' experiences of epidural pain relief during normal labour.

Defining variables

The variables and the terms contained in the hypothesis or research question must be defined so that their meaning is clear to the researcher and to the reader of the research report. Two kinds of definition are generally required:
1   A dictionary or conceptual definition.
2   An operational definition.

In a **conceptual definition**, a set of concepts defines another concept. The definition conveys the general theoretical meaning of the concept, and uses words to describe its properties. Thus, 'a hungry person' could be conceptually defined as someone who needs food, and 'post-operative pain' can be described as the discomfort that an individual experiences after a surgical procedure.

A conceptual definition cannot be true or false, but it may or may not be useful for communication in the research report. To be useful, a conceptual definition should
■   denote the distinctive characteristics of that which is defined; for example the distinctive characteristic of a hungry person is his/her need for food

- not describe something by using the same concept; for example post-operative pain should not be defined as the pain a patient experiences after an operation
- be explicit and clearly phrased to avoid different interpretations; for example defining a substance as being a drug could lead to the differing interpretations of the substance being medicinal or narcotic
- encompass all aspects of the idea that the researcher wishes to convey
- be meaningful and have meaning within the particular theoretical context
- reflect the theory used in the study
- be appropriate to and for the study, rather than simply being a term copied from a dictionary
- be consistent with common usage, literature and practice.

A conceptual definition must be professionally useful in order to be meaningful to anyone with whom the researcher wishes to communicate.

While a conceptual definition conveys the researcher's perspective on a given concept, it is insufficient in itself because it does not specify the *manner* in which the variable is to be observed and/or measured; that is, it does not describe the steps that the researcher must take in order to gather the required information.

Such a description is the function of the operational definition. An **operational definition** assigns meaning to a variable and describes the activities required to measure it. In other words, it describes how the variable under study is to be observed and measured. The operational definition should be so specific that, following it, another researcher replicating the study would be able to construct the measurement techniques in exactly the same way.

Using the example we also use above, Bless and Higson-Smith (2000) suggest three types of operational definitions for a hungry person, namely,

1 a person who has been deprived of food for 24 hours
2 a person who can eat a loaf of bread in less than 10 minutes
3 a person whose blood sugar is lower than a specified level.

Each of these definitions gives a precise indication of what the researcher needs to do or observe in order to identify the phenomenon – a hungry person. The researcher chooses the definition that best fits the particular situation or research for which it has been conceived.

To use another example, we operationally define the concept of 'obesity' as a body mass index (BMI) above 30 kilograms per square meter. BMI is the weight in kilograms divided by height in square meters. This definition enables anyone investigating obesity to assign the same meaning to the term, because it provides specificity and direction.

An operational definition may be influenced by the unavailability of direct information or the need for information to be obtained through secondary sources.

Furthermore, such a definition may be unique to a particular situation or research for which it has been formulated. For example, if the researcher is unable to assess the social status of the research subjects, he/she can determine it by observing traits such as employment level, educational level, income, material possessions and area of residence.

Research proposal

Sometimes also referred to as 'research protocol', the research proposal is a written statement or plan of the research design which the researcher must submit in order to gain approval for the study to proceed. It presents the project plan to reviewers to show them that the researcher is capable of successfully conducting the proposed research. With it, the researcher can also obtain permission for postgraduate registration at a tertiary education institution or obtain the funds needed for the study.

The ethics committees, supervisors, managers of institutions or colleagues scrutinise the proposal for methodological or ethical problems. Once they have accepted the proposal, the researcher may begin the data collection process. While the proposal shows how the research will be conducted, this is not an inflexible procedure; it can be adjusted if new insights are acquired during the research, particularly in qualitative research.

The proposal must show the reviewer that the study is based on theory; that it is methodologically sound, practically organised and logical; and that it will contribute significantly to the knowledge base of the field of interest. The compilation of the proposal also helps the researcher to clarify and refine the research process itself.

The way in which the proposal is organised under specific headings will vary, but the elements are fairly common. The actual headings are thus less important than addressing the 'what', 'why', 'how', 'who', 'where' and 'when' aspects of the study. Every aspect must be clearly worded, and provide the relevant facts in a concise, logical and systematic manner.

Du Plooy (2001: 92) suggests that the researcher asks him-/herself these 10 questions when writing a research proposal:

1 What will I research?
2 Why am I undertaking the research study?
3 What are the aims and objectives of the study?
4 What are the research questions or hypotheses?
5 What are the ethical implications?
6 How will I collect the research data?
7 Who will be involved?
8 Where will I conduct the study?
9 When will I conduct the study?
10 How will I interpret the data?

The following is an example of a proposal outline. As a researcher, you can adjust it according to the type of study or the specific requirements for obtaining permission to commence the study.

The outline of a proposal should comprise these basic elements:
- Personal details of the researcher.
- Proposed title of the study.
- Introduction, containing an overview of the broader topic or area of interest to contextualise the study.
- Background, providing an introduction to the more detailed discussion of the research problem and questions, including the rationale for the study and some literature review on the topic.
- Aim and objectives, including the problem statement.
- Demarcation of the field of study.
- Research methodology, including the design, population and sample, data collection and data analysis.
- Significance, thus persuading the reviewer of the value and importance of the study.
- Ethical considerations.
- Potential limitations.
- Project outline, including the resources that are available and those that are needed to conduct the study, as well as the organisational plan, the work plan, the schedule and the financial plan.
- Bibliography.

The research proposal forms an integral part of the research process. A good research proposal serves as the working document for the study.

Summary

In this chapter, we focused on the transformation of a broad, general problem into more manageable, researchable problems. We explored the process of stating the purpose of the study and formulating objectives, questions or hypotheses. Having addressed the identification and definition of different types of variables, we explained the preparation of a research proposal and its significance as the initial step in the broader research process.

Exercises

Complete these exercises:

1 Select and read a research article from a research journal. Then answer the following questions:
   a) Is the research problem formulated as a question, an objective or a hypothesis?
   b) Is the purpose of the study clearly stated? What is it?
   c) Does the research problem have independent and dependent variables?
   d) Are the variables operationally defined?
2 Identify any extraneous variables in your chosen article. Suggest ways of controlling these variables.
3 In the following statements, identify the independent and dependent variables:
   a) The job turnover rate and job dissatisfaction levels of graduate health care professionals who have worked less than two years is higher than for those who have worked more than two years.
   b) There is an inverse relationship between the number of prenatal classes attended by pregnant women and the degree of fear concerning giving birth.
   c) Unmarried pregnant teenagers have lower levels of self-esteem than do married pregnant teenagers.
4 Formulate an operational definition for each of these variables: pain, stress and compliance.
5 Select a research topic and draft a research proposal seeking permission to do the study.
6 Explain the importance of a research proposal.

8

Quantitative research

LEARNING OUTCOMES

On completion of this chapter, you should be able to demonstrate your understanding of

■ the relationship of the research design to the research question

■ basic research designs used in quantitative research

■ the key elements of experimental and non-experimental research designs

■ common problems, or risks to validity, inherent in the various types of research designs

■ research designs in epidemiological studies

■ the criteria for evaluating quantitative research designs.

Introduction

The focus of this chapter is on the most common types of quantitative research designs. The research design flows directly from the particular research question or hypothesis and from the specific purpose of the study. Simply stated, the research design is the set of logical steps taken by the researcher to answer the research question. It forms the 'blueprint' of the study and determines the methodology used by the researcher to obtain sources of information, such as subjects, elements and units of analysis, to collect and analyse the data, and to interpret the results.

Theoretically, with every research question there is one research design that may be considered the most appropriate to maximise the validity of the research findings. However, researchers should not lose sight of the fact that the best theoretical design might prove to be impractical or even impossible in a given situation. Researchers generally choose the design that best fits their purpose and is compatible with the resources available to them, such as time, money, sources of information and ethical considerations, and their personal preferences.

Classification of research designs

Many ways have been proposed to classify and describe research designs. Unfortunately, no single classification is entirely satisfactory. Furthermore, the same terms are often defined differently by different writers, making it difficult for the researcher to choose from each classification the one that is most useful. In Chapter 1 we discuss examples of these differences. In this chapter, we present designs under the two broad categories of quantitative and qualitative designs, which is the current trend in the health sciences literature. See Table 1.3 in Chapter 1, in which we provide the distinguishing features of quantitative and qualitative research. We discuss quantitative designs here, and non-traditional and qualitative designs in Chapter 9.

Quantitative designs can be divided into experimental and non-experimental designs, as summarised in Table 8.1 on the next page.

Experimental designs

These differ from non-experimental designs primarily in that the researcher can control the action of the specific variables being studied. The researcher manipulates the action of the independent or causal variable(s), and observes and measures the action or outcome on the dependent variable(s).

Experiments are concerned with testing hypotheses and establishing causality. Clinical practice often requires evidence generated from experimental research. Many factors, however, limit the extent to which purely experimental designs can be used in health sciences research, most notably the human nature of the subjects and the naturalistic setting. Studying human beings usually limits the researcher's control over the independent and extraneous variables involved.

Table 8.1 Quantitative designs		
Experimental	**Non-experimental**	**Non-traditional**
True experimental designs Pre-test–post-test control group designs Post-test-only control group Solomon four-group designs Factorial designs Quasi-experimental designs Time-series designs Pre-experimental designs One-shot case study One-group pre-test post-test	Descriptive designs Survey designs Simple survey Longitudinal survey Developmental survey Comparative designs Correlation designs *Ex post facto* designs Retrospective Prospective Path analysis Predictive	Case studies Historical studies Methodological studies Meta-analysis Secondary analysis Evaluation Needs assessment Action studies Philosophical studies

Source: Based on Nieswiadomy (1993: 128) and Talbot (1995: 217–39)

True experimental designs

In order for the experiment to qualify as true, three conditions are necessary:

1 **Manipulation.** The term 'manipulation' signifies that the independent variable, which may be an event, an intervention or a treatment that he/she expects will have an effect on the dependent variable, is controlled by the researcher. In other words, the researcher manipulates the independent variable to assess or measure its impact on the dependent variable. For example, the researcher could introduce an intervention, such as an educational programme or a treatment, to some subjects and withhold it from others. He/she then observes the effect of the intervention or lack thereof. He/she decides what is to be manipulated, for example the type of educational programme, to whom the manipulation applies, when the manipulation is to occur and how the manipulation is to be implemented.

2 **Control.** The researcher must be able to exercise control in the experimental situation by eliminating the actions of other variables beyond the independent ones. He/she can achieve this control by manipulating, randomising, blocking, matching and carefully preparing experimental protocols, and by using control groups. In other words, the researcher imposes rules to decrease the possibility of error and increase the likelihood that the research findings are an accurate reflection of the effect of the intervention.

3 **Randomisation.** A true experimental design requires that the researcher is able to assign subjects to the experimental or control groups on a random basis. Random assignment means that each subject has an equal chance of being put in any of the treatment groups. The assumption is that if this is done, the differences in the groups will be owing to the manipulation of the independent variables, and not to different characteristics in the subjects that the researcher has not measured and may not even know about.

    To achieve randomisation, the researcher first identifies the entire, accessible group of subjects, then randomly divides this group into two or more subgroups, depending on the chosen design, through the use of random number tables, coin flipping or certain other techniques, which we explore in Chapter 10.

We now explore the basic true experimental designs.

Pre-test–post-test control group design

In this design, subjects are randomly assigned to two groups, namely, the experimental group and the control group. Both groups are measured at the beginning of the study in a pre-test. Then the experimental group is subjected to the event or intervention, after which both groups are measured again. The researcher can now compare the pre-test and post-test scores of the experimental group, as well as the post-test scores of the control group, in order to assess whether the event or intervention made any difference to the scores of the experimental group.

    Figure 8.1 illustrates this design.

Time line of study events				
	Randomisation	Pre-test	Experiment	Post-test
Groups Experimental Control	R R	01 01	× –	02 02
0 = Dependent variable measured × = Application of independent variable R = Random assignment – = no intervention				

Figure 8.1 Pre-test–post-test control group design

For example, a researcher is interested in the usefulness of an educational video on diabetes. He/she randomly assigns diabetic patients to experimental and control groups and pre-tests both groups on their knowledge of diabetes. The experimental group then watches the educational video, while the control group is given written information similar to that covered in the video. Both groups are then post-tested on their knowledge of diabetes. Finally, the researcher compares the difference between the post-test scores of the two groups.

Owing to randomisation, it is expected that the two groups will be equivalent at the pre-test phase. But it is possible that they may differ, in which case the researcher takes the difference in the pre-test into account when comparing the post-test results. This design allows the researcher to measure the effects of history, maturation and regression on the mean, which we discuss in more detail later in this chapter.

Post-test-only control group design

In this design there is no pre-test, as illustrated in Figure 8.2. The design is particularly useful in situations in which it is not possible to obtain a pre-test measure. In many studies it may be inappropriate or impossible to pre-test before the independent variable is manipulated. For example, a researcher wishes to study the effect of a particular intervention on the incidence of post-operative vomiting following cholecystectomy. It would be inappropriate to develop and induce a pre-test of vomiting behaviour. However, a random sample of cholecystectomy patients undergoing the same medical treatment and anaesthesia could be randomly assigned to control and experimental groups, and their possible post-operative vomiting could be tested.

	Randomisation	Experiment	Post-test
Groups Experimental Control	R R	× –	01 01

Figure 8.2 Post-test-only control group design

Solomon four-group design

This design combines the two preceding designs, and is illustrated in Figure 8.3 on the next page. Subjects are randomly selected from the population, then randomly assigned to four groups. Two groups receive pre-tests and two groups do not. Administering a pre-test may in itself have some influence on the outcome of the experiment, that is, the post-test scores. By combining the pre-test–post-test control group design with the post-test-only control group design to form the Solomon four-group design, the researcher can control the effect of the pre-test.

	Randomisation	Pre-test	Experiment	Post-test
Groups				
1 Experimental	R	01	×	02
2 Control	R	01	–	02
3 Experimental	R		×	01
4 Control	R		–	01

Figure 8.3 Solomon four-group design

This is considered to be an extremely powerful experimental design because it mini-mises threats to internal and external validity and controls for the reaction effects of the pre-test. Any differences between the pre-test–post-test groups and the post-test-only groups can be more confidently associated with the experimental intervention.

The design is frequently used in health sciences research to study various combinations of interventions. However, possible disadvantages are that it requires a large sample and the statistical analysis of the data is complicated.

Randomised clinical trials

The randomised clinical trial (RCT) is a type of experimental design that intends to evaluate the efficacy of intervention and to establish a reliable cause–effect relationship. This design is characterised by the following:

- **Selection criteria.** To ensure that the groups are comparable on all the characteristics that might influence the outcome of the study, groups are selected according to pre-specified inclusion and exclusion criteria.
- **Random sampling.** To ensure that all the potential subjects have an equal chance of being included in either the experimental or the control group, random sampling is done as the first level of sampling, before random assignment to groups.
- **Control.** The researcher introduces control of the experimental situation to eliminate threats to validity, using one or more controls. One control is to use a control group that has been assigned through the process of randomisation.
- **Double-blind procedure.** Neither the researcher nor the subjects should know to which group the subjects have been assigned.
- **Intervention protocol.** To ensure that each subject receives the intervention in exactly the same way, intervention procedures are standardised.
- **Crossover design.** Subjects could be re-assigned to the other intervention in the trial and the responses to the different interventions are then compared.
- **Intention-to-treat analysis.** The responses of subjects are analysed within their group.
- **Effect size.** Intervention and non-intervention outcomes are compared.

To increase the sample size and the resources, clinical trials may be carried out simultaneously in multiple geographical locations – these are the so-called 'multi-centred RCTs'. Randomised clinical trials do not take place in the laboratory setting but in the clinical environment, for example the effect of Aloe Vera gel/mild soap versus mild soap alone in preventing skin reactions in patients undergoing radiation therapy (Olsen et al. 2001). (Oncology Nursing Forum: 543–47).

Factorial design

Factorial designs allow the researcher to test the effect of more than one independent variable in the same experiment simultaneously. The independent variables are referred to as 'factors' and both their individual and combined effects can be measured. Typical factorial designs usually incorporate a 2 × 2 factorial, or a 3 × 3 factorial, but any combination is possible. The first number refers to the independent variables and the second number to the levels of intervention, as illustrated in Figure 8.4. For example, types of therapy – individual counselling (y1) or group counselling (y2) – can be factors, and lengths of intervention – brief counselling (x1), intermediate counselling (x2) or long-term counselling (x3) – can be levels of intervention. This would yield a 2 × 3 factorial design, and subjects would be randomly assigned to one of the six combinations, or cells, that would result from this design.

	x1	x2	x3
y1	x1 y1	x2 y2	x3 y1
y2	x1 y2	x2 y2	x3 y2

Figure 8.4 Factorial design

In the above example, the researcher could determine whether long-term individual counselling is more effective than short-term counselling, or which type of counselling – individual or group – is most effective.

Quasi-experimental designs

In real life, it is often difficult for the researcher to obtain a control group either by randomisation or by matching. These difficulties introduce the need for the relaxation of some of the requirements of the true experiment. For example, the researcher may omit a control group for comparison, or, if he/she uses a control group, he/she may omit randomisation in sampling and assignment to experimental and control groups. In other words, the researcher uses a quasi-experimental design. Within the context of this design, the control group is often referred to as a 'comparison group'.

There are many quasi-experimental designs outlined in the research literature. We discuss two of the most frequently encountered designs.

Non-equivalent control group design

This is the most basic and widely used design in health sciences research. It is similar to the pre-test–post-test control group design, except that there is no random assignment of subjects to experimental and comparison groups. Instead, the researcher selects two similar available groups. For example, he/she chooses a group of diabetics attending Diabetic Out-patients Clinic A and another group attending Diabetic Out-patients Clinic B. The experimental intervention is administered to one group, the experimental group, while the comparison group would receive no intervention, or an alternative intervention. The biggest threat to internal validity in this design is *selection bias* (see further below). The two groups may have been dissimilar at the beginning of the study; it is possible, however, to test statistically for differences in the group. Babbie and Mouton (2001) point out that it is better to use a non-equivalent control group than no comparison group at all.

Time-series design

In this design, the researcher collects data on the dependent variable from the experimental group at set intervals, both before and after the introduction of the independent variable. No control group is used for comparison. The data collected prior to and after the introduction of the independent variable are compared for differences in the dependent variable. For example, the researcher assesses the pain levels of a group of patients with lower back pain. After three weeks of pain assessment (01, 02, 03), subjects could be taught a particular exercise to alleviate the lower back pain. During the next three weeks, pain levels would again be measured (04, 05, 06). The results of this study help the researcher to determine if the lower back pain persists, if the exercise is effective in reducing the pain, and, if so, whether the efficacy persists.

The strength of this design lies in the repeated data collection over periods of time before and after the introduction of the independent variable. Subjects act as their own control, providing a strong indication that the independent variable could be responsible for observed change in the dependent variable.

Pre-experimental designs

These are designs that are weak, and in which the researcher has little control over the research. At times these designs are provided as examples of how *not* to do research (Nieswiadomy 1993). Included among these designs arc once-off case studies and one-group pre-test–post-test designs.

Problems with experimental designs

Although experimental designs are effective in explaining cause–effect relationships between variables, they are subject to the following limitations that make them difficult to apply to many real-world problems:

■ A number of interesting variables simply are not amenable to experimental manipulation. For example, the researcher cannot manipulate health history, or subjects' age or gender.

■ Many variables can be manipulated, but ethical considerations prohibit this. For example, it would be unethical for the researcher to withhold treatment from a patient, or to expose him/her to danger.

■ Experimental designs simply may not be feasible; they may require additional funds and be difficult to conduct in natural settings such as hospitals or clinics.

■ Experiments are complicated by many sources of bias and errors – threats to internal and external validity – which must be dealt with as effectively as possible to ensure that the research is of a high quality. The researcher must always contend with competing explanations for the obtained results.

Threats to internal validity

'Internal validity' refers to the degree to which the outcomes of an experiment can be attributed to the manipulated, independent variable(s) rather than to uncontrolled extraneous factors. Other than the independent variable, any factor that influences the dependent variable constitutes a threat to validity.

Babbie and Mouton (2001), and Burns and Grove (2003), have identified several threats to the internal validity of a study:

■ **History.** This refers to events, other than the experimental intervention, which occur during the course of a study – between pre-test and post-test – and which might affect the results. For example, in a study of the effects of an exercise programme on hypertension, some of the patients might take up additional exercise, such as tennis, which may have an effect on the outcome. In a study of the effects of compulsory community service of newly graduated health care professionals on the quality of patient care, factors such as staffing changes, new policies or changes in patient intake may have profound effects on the quality of care.

History is controlled by the use of at least one simultaneous comparison group. Additionally, random assignment of subjects to groups will help to control the threat of history. In the form of extraneous events, history would therefore be as likely to occur in one group as in another. A time-series design may also help to reduce the effect of unanticipated events on, or normal fluctuations in, the dependent variables.

■ **Maturation.** This refers to changes that occur within subjects over time, which may affect experimental results. These changes include physical growth, the mastering of new developmental skills, intellectual maturity, normal healing following an injury or illness, or stress and anxiety. In general, the longer the experimental intervention, the more difficult it is to rule out the effects of maturation. The one-group pre-test–post-test design is particularly vulnerable to this threat.

- **Testing.** One of the difficulties inherent in research utilising a pre-test–post-test design is the effect of testing and re-testing. Prior exposure to a test or measurement technique can bias a subject's responses. He/she may remember previous inaccurate responses and have the desire to change these, which would alter the outcome of the study. Particular test effects are boredom – when exactly the same test is repeated, practice – as subjects learn through repetition to respond to tests, and fatigue – particularly when the test is lengthy. In order to counter these effects, the researcher should reduce the number of times that subjects are tested, vary the tests slightly to reduce boredom and practice effects, and use shorter tests to reduce fatigue. The Solomon four-group design counters the effect of pre-tests.

- **Instrumentation.** Instruments may present a threat to validity particularly when those used to record measurements change over time. The changes can occur when humans are the instrument, or when different instruments, physical equipment or measuring scales are utilised. Human observers can gain experience and become more proficient in their ratings, or, by contrast, may become tired and make less exact observations. Equipment can record inaccurate readings and, with repeated use, may need to be recalibrated to maintain accuracy of measurement.

- **Mortality.** Frequently, subjects may drop out of a study during the data-collection procedures. There may be more dropouts in one group than in others, causing the groups to differ. It is also possible that the subjects who drop out are systematically different from those who remain, and this may result in biased findings. For example, if a large number of experimental group subjects who score very low on the pre-test drop out, the average scores on the post-test for the experimental group may be deceptively high. The researcher should design the study so that it is convenient for the subjects to participate until the end, and should impress upon them the importance of their continuing cooperation.

- **Selection bias.** Selection becomes a problem when differences exist in the way that subjects are recruited for a study and assigned to groups. Unless subjects in each group can be shown to be similar *before* the intervention, the researcher will have difficulty attributing causality to the experimental intervention. It is therefore important that the researcher takes steps to ensure that the subjects in all intervention groups are as similar as possible. Random selection and assignment or matching decreases the potential for selection to be a threat to validity.

■ **Demoralisation.** A feeling of deprivation may occur in the control group when subjects realise that they are receiving less desirable interventions. They may withdraw, give up or become angry. These behaviours are *reactions to* the intervention, and not *caused by* the intervention. They can lead to differences that are not attributable to the intervention.

Threats to external validity

'External validity' refers to the degree to which the results of a study can be generalised to other people and other settings. Questions to be answered about external validity are as follows:

■ With what degree of confidence can the study findings be transferred from the sample to the entire population?

■ Will these findings hold true in other times and places?

The researcher needs to consider several threats to external validity:

■ **Reactive effects.** These are a group of related effects resulting from the fact that the subjects know that they are being observed and thus behave in an unnatural manner. An example of a reactive effect is test anxiety. The measuring instrument may increase the arousal levels of some subjects and thus influence their scores. Similarly, certain subjects try to please the researcher and provide the results that they believe are desired. Others will do just the opposite, and try to confound the study in order to find out how the researcher will react.

■ **Researcher effects.** These threaten the study results when researcher characteristics or behaviour influence the subjects' behaviour. Examples of influential researcher characteristics or behaviour are verbal or non-verbal cues, facial expressions, clothing, age and gender. Researchers may also exert bias in recording observations in a way that produces more favourable results. A useful way to control for this effect is for the researcher to remain 'blind' to group assignments; that is, the researcher is unaware which is the experimental group and which is the control group. If both the researcher and the subjects remain unaware of group assignment, we know that double blinding has been employed.

The **Hawthorne effect** may be a threat to *both* external and internal validity. It occurs when subjects respond in a certain manner because they are aware that they are being observed. The most effective way of countering this source of bias is to use unobtrusive techniques of data collection. In other words, if the subjects are not aware that they are being observed, there is no reason for them to act unusually and, more importantly, no reason for the researcher to *expect* them to do so. Of course, this is not always possible, particularly in light of the necessity of obtaining informed consent. In other cases, the researcher should collect data in a way that causes the least disturbance to the subjects' lives. In practice, this may mean collecting facts in the subjects' daily environments, and using techniques that do not require special skills or unusual apparatus. The onus, however, is on the researcher to show that the effect is caused by the intervention and not simply by the subjects' participation in the study.

Non-experimental designs

Non-experimental designs are clearly distinguishable from true experimental and quasi-experimental designs in that there is no manipulation of the independent variable and, therefore, no intervention; nor is the setting controlled. The study is carried out in a natural setting and phenomena are observed as they occur. The major purpose of non-experimental research is to describe phenomena, and explore and explain the relationships between variables. The lack of experimental control makes these designs less able to determine cause and effect than true or quasi-experiments, but they are highly useful in generating knowledge in a variety of situations in which it is difficult, unethical or even impossible to employ an experimental approach. Variables that are difficult to manipulate, or the manipulation of which is unethical, include pain, social support, fear, obesity, alcohol intake, drug abuse, grieving, and physical or emotional illness. It is as important for the researcher to obtain valid study results in non-experimental research as it is in experimental research. Thus, the researcher needs to consider the extraneous variables that threaten the validity of non-experimental studies.

While many types of non-experimental designs are described in the literature, there are two broad categories.

Descriptive designs

These are used in studies where more information is required in a particular field through the provision of a picture of the phenomenon as it occurs naturally. These designs describe the variables in order to answer the research question, and there is no intention of establishing a cause–effect relationship. Descriptive research encompasses a wide variety of designs that utilise both quantitative and qualitative methods.

According to Brink and Wood (1998), descriptive designs are based on the following assumptions:

- The variable exists in the study population as a single variable that is amenable to description.
- There is insufficient existing literature describing the study population or the variable.
- The study may commence without a theoretical framework but the researcher should provide the rationale for the study based on a thorough literature review.

- Existing studies may provide the rationale and theoretical framework for the study at hand, in the case of a known concept.
- In a study where the criteria for external validity cannot be met owing to unknown population parameters, the findings cannot be generalised.

Descriptive designs are concerned with gathering information from a representative sample of the population. The emphasis in the collection of data in descriptive studies is on structured observation, questionnaires and interviews or survey studies.

Figure 8.5 illustrates the manner in which the researcher can determine the most suitable type of study design.

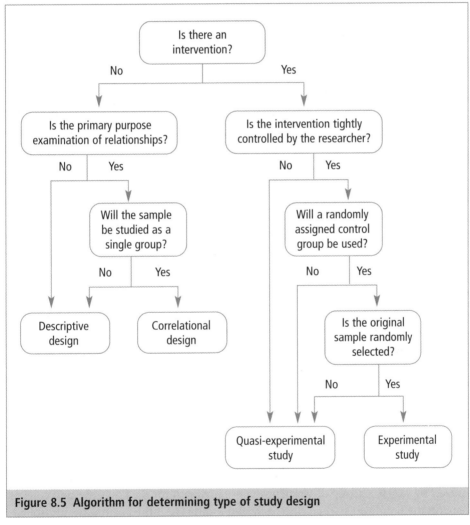

Figure 8.5 Algorithm for determining type of study design

Source: Adapted from Burns and Grove (2003: 201)

Typical descriptive study

This is intended merely to describe a phenomenon. The researcher does not manipulate any variables, and makes no effort to determine the relationship between variables. In these studies, the researcher merely searches for accurate information about the characteristics of a single sample – subjects, groups, institutions or situations – or about the frequency of a phenomenon's occurrence. He/she should identify and conceptually and operationally define the variables of interest. These variables can be classified as opinions, attitudes, needs or facts, after which they are described to provide a complete picture of the phenomenon as it exists.

An example of an opinion or attitude variable is the responses of health care professionals at different educational levels to abortion. An example of a descriptive study focusing on needs is the examination of the psychological needs of individuals diagnosed with Aids. An example of variables that are facts is the percentage of teenage mothers who receive inadequate antenatal care.

Comparative descriptive study

A comparative descriptive study is designed to describe variables as well as the differences between or among two or more groups to see if they differ on some variable. Descriptive and inferential statistics may be used to analyse these differences. For example, a researcher wants to investigate the level of self-esteem of abused children. He/she chooses a group of children who have experienced abuse and compares them with a group of children who have not been abused to see to what extent they differ with regard to self-esteem. Another researcher is interested in studying the effect of widowhood on physical and psychological well-being. He/she proceeds by taking two groups as they naturally occur, that is, widows and married people, comparing them in terms of physical and psychological well-being, and providing detailed descriptive information about them.

Descriptive designs with a time dimension

The researcher plans and conducts a study with a **longitudinal** design when he/she wishes to examine the way in which variables change over time. In other words, this design uses a time perspective. The researcher is concerned not only with the existing status and interrelationship of phenomena, but also with changes that result from significantly elapsed time.

Longitudinal studies allow the researcher to collect data at several points in time. For instance, a midwife is interested in investigating the development of maternal bonding with the unborn baby in relation to the first time the mother felt the baby move. She selects a group of women who are pregnant for the first time, and collects data on the bonding process from each of the subjects at the twelfth, twenty-fourth and thirty-sixth week of pregnancy. This provides a longitudinal perspective of the bonding process. This example can be seen as a short-term longitudinal study. In some instances, longitudinal studies are long term and can continue for years. Particularly if they stretch over the long term, longitudinal studies are expensive and require ongoing subject and researcher commitment. There are also many threats to validity that must be taken into account.

Cross-sectional studies are used to examine data at one point in time, that is, the data are collected on one occasion only with different subjects, rather than on the same subjects at several points in time. For example, the midwife conducting the above study now selects equivalent groups of women who are pregnant for the first time and who are at each of the respective points of pregnancy; that is, she collects data from a group of subjects who are 12 weeks pregnant, from another but equivalent group who are 24 weeks pregnant, and from yet another equivalent group who are 36 weeks pregnant. She then compares the data from each group using statistical measures.

Correlational design

This is also known as '*ex post facto*' or 'after the fact' design. Its basic purposes are to describe existing relationships between variables, and to determine the relationship between independent and dependent variables. When a correlation exists, a change in one variable corresponds to a change in others.

In correlational studies, there is no manipulation of the independent variable, because the event of interest, or the dependent variable, has already occurred. Therefore, it is clear that correlation does not indicate causation. This type of research may confirm the existence of a correlation, but it is generally insufficient to indicate that a causal relationship exists.

In descriptive correlational design, the researcher attempts to determine and describe the relationships existing between variables. For example, a researcher wishes to study the relationship between age and body weight. As it is impossible to manipulate age, the researcher records the body weight of subjects from a variety of age groups. He/she then determines the relationship between age and body weight statistically through the use of a statistical test known as the 'correlation coefficient'.

When using a **retrospective design**, the researcher starts with an effect and works backwards to determine what was associated with this effect in the past. An example is the thalidomide babies: when large numbers of birth defects – armless and legless babies – were reported in the 1960s, researchers started looking backwards for factors that might have been the cause or that might be correlated with the effect. They found that all the mothers of these babies had taken thalidomide, a sedative, during pregnancy. Hence, researchers could establish a relationship between the drug and specific birth defects.

In a **prospective study**, the researcher selects a population and follows it over time to determine outcomes. For example, a researcher wants to study the impact of arthritis – pain and functional impairment – on the quality of life. He selects a group of arthritis patients and determines their pain and functional impairment. He follows up the cases over a period of time to determine the subjects' quality of life.

The value of correlational designs lies in the fact that many important research problems cannot be studied by experimentation. Moreover, correlational designs are usually inexpensive, they can be done quickly, they can use large samples from a given population, and they can provide meaningful information about how variables function in relation to one another.

Epidemiological research

Epidemiology is concerned with all health and illness in the human population, and with the factors, including health services, that affect them. **Epidemiological research** involves the gathering of information on disease/health in groups of people, and on agents causing change or preventing disease or recovery in the environment.

When doing epidemiological research, the researcher must pose the following questions:

■ Why has this person rather than another developed a specific disease?
■ How could a specific disease be prevented?
■ Why does a specific disease occur in one season rather than in another?
■ Why is a disease more prevalent in this country than in another?

Epidemiological descriptive studies consist of the description of patterns of disease in populations, and involve the measurement of mortality, morbidity and disability. Other typical epidemiological research includes case-control studies, cohort studies, randomised clinical trials, meta-analysis, longitudinal and cross-sectional studies, and correlational studies. The main uses of epidemiological studies in health sciences comprise

■ the investigation of the causes and natural history of disease with the aim of prevention and health promotion
■ the measurement of health care needs and the evaluation of clinical management with the aim of improving the efficacy and efficiency of health care
■ the development of risk screening and diagnostic instruments.

In short, epidemiological findings play a *major* role in clinical decision-making and the development of health care policies.

Evaluating quantitative research designs

Evidently, the designs we discuss have significant strengths and a number of problems. In evaluating a published research report, as a researcher you may experience difficulty in deciding which aspects of the design make the study useful and important, and which aspects imply flaws that inhibit the use of the findings in practice. Table 8.2 presents a summary of several criteria that you can use when evaluating a research design.

Table 8.2 Evaluation criteria for research design	
1	Which specific type of design is used in the study?
2	Is the design appropriate for the research question?
3	Is the design congruent with the purpose of the study?
4	Given the nature of the research question, what type of design is most appropriate? How much flexibility does the research question require, and how much structure is needed? Was this provided for?
5	Is the design suited to the data-collection method?
6	Are the research methods clearly described?
7	How well does the research design control or account for threats to internal and external validity?
8	What threats to validity are not controlled by the research design? How does this affect the usefulness of the results?
9	How well does the research design determine causality between dependent and independent variables?

Summary

In this chapter, we presented an overview of the most common quantitative designs found in health sciences research, namely, experimental designs, quasi-experimental designs and non-experimental descriptive and correlational designs. We discussed the threats to internal and external validity that a researcher must always take into consideration and attempt to control. We closed the chapter with a summary of the criteria for evaluating a research design, which is directed towards assessing the suitability of the selected design in relation to factors such as the research question and purpose, the methodology and confounding variables.

Exercises

Complete these exercises:

1 Answer the following questions based on your knowledge of the types of research design we present in the chapter:
   a) What features characterise each type?
   b) In what ways do the major research designs differ from one another?
   c) What are the strengths and limitations of each type of research design?
   d) List specific research questions that could be explored with regard to each type of design.
2 Imagine that you want to test the following hypothesis: 'Health care practitioner efficacy is higher in primary health care than in team health care'. Answer these related questions:
   a) What research design is appropriate for this study?
   b) What are the potential threats to validity in using the chosen research design?
   c) How could you, as the researcher, reduce bias in the study?

9

Non-traditional and qualitative research designs

LEARNING OUTCOMES

On completion of this chapter, you should be able to demonstrate your understanding of

- the purposes and some of the distinguishing features of non-traditional designs
- the aims of qualitative research
- the areas in health sciences research where qualitative approaches are particularly useful
- the key elements common to various qualitative research designs
- the nature and function of phenomenology, ethnography, grounded theory and philosophy
- the validity and reliability (trustworthiness) of qualitative research designs
- the relationship of the research design to the research purpose.

Introduction

In the previous chapter, we provided a broad overview of traditional quantitative designs. In this chapter, we continue the discussion with regard to non-traditional and qualitative designs. There is some discrepancy in the literature about the categorisation of non-traditional designs. For the purpose of this book we use the terms that are used in health sciences research, but which do not fit easily into either the experimental or non-experimental categories.

Non-traditional designs

Case studies

A case study is an in-depth study of an individual, a group of individuals or an institution. For example, a health sciences researcher could study how one of his/her diabetic patients responds to an insulin pump. Another researcher could examine an institution for the dying, such as a hospice. Case studies are frequently used when there is a new phenomenon about which little is known, or rare events in which few subjects can be found. Case studies provide significant amounts of descriptive information, and they can also present explanatory information; in other words, they can explain the causes of the phenomenon or event in addition to describing it, therefore studying the *why* and *what*.

Researchers conducting case studies use a number of approaches to the collection and analysis of data. Popular approaches include questionnaires, interviews, observations and written accounts by the subjects. The disadvantages of case studies are that they tend to be time-consuming and quite costly, and subject drop-out may occur if the study is carried out over an extended period. The advantage is the detailed level of analysis that results when research is confined to a small number of subjects.

Historical research

In historical research, researchers study past events. However, historical research should not be confused with *ex post facto* research in which a retrospective design is used. The focus of the two is usually quite different. Historical research involves a detailed study and analysis of individuals, events, institutions or specific time periods. The purpose is to gain a clearer understanding of the impact of the past on present and future events.

Historical research generally involves the review of written materials, but it may encompass oral documentation as well. Diaries, letters, manuscripts, maps and books are but a few of the documents that may be considered. The documents should be original or primary sources wherever possible. Once the data has been collected, it should be subjected to two types of evaluation: external and internal criticism. **External** criticism is concerned with the authenticity or genuine nature of the data, and **internal criticism** examines the accuracy of the data. While the former establishes the *validity* of the data, the latter establishes the *reliability* of the data. The researcher's use of original authentic sources, his/her awareness of his/her own bias, and the substantiation of the document in question by another collaborating source are some of the safeguards that the researcher uses to ensure that his/her interpretations are correct.

Methodological research

Methodological studies focus on the development, testing and evaluation of research instruments and methods used in research investigations. The goal is to improve the trustworthiness (reliability and validity) of data-collection tools.

Meta-analysis

In a meta-analysis, the results from a large number of existing studies, that had been scrutinised for methodology and quality, are used as one piece of data for statistical analysis, quantitatively summarising the findings. A meta-analysis is usually done on a particular topic, for example pain management. The researcher consults the published literature for relevant studies and the results of each of these studies become one piece of data (unit of analysis).

Evaluation research

The purpose of evaluation research is to find out how well a programme, treatment or practice policy concerning an intervention is implemented, how well it accomplishes its purpose, and how useful it is. There are three broad categories of evaluation research: diagnostic, formative and summative evaluation. **Diagnostic evaluation** research may help the people who are implementing an intervention to identify the neglected areas of need and problems within programmes or organisations. **Formative evaluation** of an existing programme or intervention determines whether it was implemented as planned, whether it is working as planned, and whether it can be improved. A **summative evaluation** is conducted on an ongoing or completed programme to determine whether the programme has met the stated objectives. Evaluations can employ experimental, quasi-experimental, non-experimental or qualitative designs, and can either be cross-sectional or longitudinal.

Needs assessment

As the term implies, needs assessment is a study in which a researcher collects data for estimating the needs of a group, community or organisation for certain types of services or policies. Through a survey (descriptive design) approach, the researcher can obtain direct information on the needs and perceived needs of a broad spectrum of people. For example, a health sciences researcher may wish to gather information about the supportive needs of elderly people in the community and in homes for older persons by means of a survey. Alternatively, the researcher can use the **key informant approach**, which collects information concerning the needs of a group from key individuals who are presumed to be in a position of knowledge; in other words, input is obtained from 'insiders'.

The advantage of conducting a needs assessment is that it is a useful planning tool, and the information obtained can help to establish priorities.

Action research

Fundamentally, action research is a strategy that brings about social change through action, that is, through developing and improving practice and, at the same time, generating and testing theory. Action research is a way of doing research and working on solving a problem at the same time. The researcher and the participants work together to analyse the situation that they wish to change. This may include doing some baseline measures using questionnaires, observation or other research methods. After the assessment, they plan the desired change, set their objectives and decide how to bring about the change. While they are putting their plans into action, they continue to monitor progress, changing their plans if appropriate. At the completion of the change process, they make a final assessment and draw conclusions, perhaps writing a report on the project for themselves and/or others.

Thus, action research is participatory – it encourages the active participation of the people whom the researcher intends to assist. In this way, it empowers the people to be involved in all aspects of the project, including the planning and implementation of the research and any solutions that emerge. Action research demands that the researcher and the community bring valuable resources to the project. Furthermore, this type of research is an ongoing learning process for everyone involved.

Bless and Higson-Smith (2000) point out that action research can be a particularly valuable tool in *developing countries* because it

- is concerned with solving the specific problems facing communities
- helps individuals, communities and organisations to learn skills and obtain resources so that they can function more effectively in future
- provides a way of spreading the understanding gained through research to people and communities who can benefit from those findings
- attempts to understand the person and the community within the broader social context
- aids communication between social researchers and communities in need of assistance
- shakes the 'ivory tower' of many social scientists and makes their work directly beneficial to society.

Qualitative designs

Researchers who wish to explore the meaning, or describe and promote under-standing, of human experiences such as pain, grief, hope or caring, or unfamiliar phenomena such as female genital mutilation, and so on, would find it extremely difficult to quantify the data. Qualitative methods are more appropriate and effective alternatives in such cases.

A variety of research designs falls under the umbrella of qualitative research. While each method has a specific focus and goal for discovering knowledge, there are commonalities that bind them together. As the name implies, qualitative methods focus on the qualitative aspects of meaning, experience and understanding, and they study human experience from the viewpoint of the research participants in the context in which the action takes place. We describe further characteristics in Table 1.3 of Chapter 1. We now explore the four most frequently used approaches of conducting qualitative research in the health care sciences.

Phenomenology

Phenomenological studies examine human experience through the descriptions that are provided by the people involved. The experiences are called 'lived experiences'. The purpose of phenomenological research, then, is to describe what people experience in regard to certain phenomena, as well as how they interpret the experi-ences or what meaning the experiences hold for them. Therefore, phenomenology is an approach that concentrates on a subject's experience rather than on the person as a subject or object.

In attempting to describe the lived experience, the researcher focuses on what is happening in the life of the individual, what is important about the experience and what alterations can be made. In this way, the researcher can understand, for example, what 'health' or 'caring' means to the patient. The approach may lead to the development of concepts and themes which can be applied in practice.

Like other quantitative and qualitative approaches, this approach consists of a set of steps or stages that guide researchers in the study of phenomena. While several authors have suggested the steps (Collaizi 1978; Giorgi 1970; Spiegelberg 1976; Van Kaam 1969 and Van Manen 1990), you should note that they are not fixed, and can vary from study to study.

There are certain basic actions that the researcher uses during the enquiry process:

- **Bracketing.** In this process, the researcher identifies and sets aside any preconceived beliefs and opinions that he/she might have about the phenomenon under investigation; in other words, the researcher identifies what he/she expects to discover and then deliberately sets aside this idea. The researcher 'brackets out' any preconceived ideas so that he/she can consider every available perspective.

■ **Intuiting.** This occurs when the researcher tries to develop an awareness of the lived experience. The process requires the researcher to become totally immersed in the phenomenon under investigation, aided by the participants' descriptions. The researcher reviews the data again and again until there is a common understanding. Analysing entails contrasting and comparing the final data to determine what patterns or themes emerge. If the knowledge is to be of relevance to other researchers, it must be understandable and clear, detailing the relationships that exist. The researcher must therefore pay careful attention to description.

The data-collection techniques include participant observation in the natural environment, in-depth or unstructured interviews, and diary recording. We discuss these further in Chapter 11.

There are many classic examples of phenomenological studies in health sciences research. Riemen, cited in Munhall and Oiler (1986), studies caring interactions in health care practitioner–patient relationships, and offers a useful example of how Collaizi's procedural steps can be followed. Other examples are Anderson's (1991) study of the existential experience of illness in a group of immigrant women, Rose's (1990) study of women's inner strength, Santopinto's (1989) study of the drive to be thinner, and a study of living with addiction by Banonis (1989).

Ethnography

Ethnography is a qualitative approach that grew out of social anthropology and the study of the culture and customs of groups of people. The focus of ethnography is the social and cultural world of a particular group. An underlying assumption is that the behaviour of people can only be understood within the cultural context in which it occurs. This differs from phenomenology, which focuses on the meaning of the experience rather than on the role of culture in shaping the experience.

An entire cultural group, or a subgroup in the culture, may be studied. The term 'culture' can be used in a broad sense to mean an entire tribe, for example the Masai or the Tsonga, or in a more narrow sense where it is limited to a subunit of a single institution, such as the hospital operating room, the classroom, the doctor's waiting room or a retirement village. Whatever the scope, the central aim of ethnography is to describe another way of life from the 'native' point of view (Spradley 1980). The term 'going native' was coined to describe a researcher who tries to integrate into the community he/she wishes to study and takes part in the activities in which his/her subjects engage.

In this way, the researcher is actually able to experience the world of his/her subjects – a phenomenon which is described as 'emic'. The researcher operating from the **emic perspective** examines the language of the culture, learns the organising frameworks and describes the cultural perception of reality from the viewpoint of a member of that culture. In other words, the researcher is able to obtain and provide the insider's view. By contrast, the **etic perspective** is the researcher's *interpretation* of the experiences of that culture. As the outsider, the researcher imposes meaning on the cultural experiences of his/her subjects.

The techniques of collecting and analysing data may vary according to the different forms of ethnography. However, the main techniques appear to be participant observation and unstructured interviews. Ethnographers interview people who are most knowledgeable about the culture. These people are commonly referred to as 'key informants'. Other relevant data sources include documents, life histories, films, photographs and artefacts. The researcher writes extensive field notes about these data sources to describe the observations he/she makes. Moreover, he/she uses qualitative content analysis to derive patterns and themes from the data, and reports the findings in a narrative form.

Many researchers have undertaken ethnographic studies. Among them are Leininger (1985), who studied the phenomenon of caring in various cultures; Kinzel (1991), who studied the health concerns of two homeless groups; Luyas (1991), who focused on diabetics among Mexican-Americans; and Villaruil (1995), who researched Mexican-Americans' experiences of pain.

There are many derivatives of ethnography. Leininger (1991: 76) has developed an interpretation of ethnography that she calls "ethnonursing" and defines it as "a research method to help nurses systematically document and gain greater understanding and meaning of people's daily life experiences related to human care, health and well-being in different or similar environmental contexts". The goal of ethnonursing is to discover nursing knowledge as known, perceived and experienced by nurses and consumers of nursing and health services.

Grounded theory

In its simplest form, this is the theory that emerges out of data grounded in the observation and interpretation of phenomena. Strauss and Corbin (1990: 24) describe the approach as "a qualitative research method that uses a systematic set of procedures to develop an inductively derived grounded theory about a phenomenon". The approach identifies concepts and the relationship between them in an inductive manner. The purpose is to build theory that is faithful to and illuminates the area under study.

As in the case of ethnography, the process begins in the social and cultural environment. Unlike ethnography, however, grounded theory does not seek to understand culture and cultural processes; rather, reality is perceived as a social construct. In grounded theory the researcher immerses him-/herself in the social environment.

The techniques of data collection are the same as in most other forms of qualitative research, namely, participant observation and unstructured interviews. Observations are made about the structure and patterns noted in the social environment and people's interactions are studied through interviews. Document analyses of organisational charts and policies, patient records and other sources of data provide additional perspectives to illuminating the social phenomenon. The researcher records the interview and observation data in handwritten notes and tape recordings.

One of the fundamental features of this approach is that data collection and data analysis occur simultaneously. A procedure called 'constant comparison' is used in which newly collected data are constantly compared to existing data so that commonalities and variations can be determined. An incident is compared with another incident, category with category and construct with construct across all observations. Significant incidents or observations are marked or highlighted in the text, and assigned codes. These codes are constantly reviewed as new interpretations are made of the data. The researcher keeps an open mind and uses an intuitive process of interpretation, a process that we describe in greater detail in Chapter 12.

Once he/she has identified concepts and specified their relationships, the researcher consults the literature to determine if any similar associations exist. Despite the great diversity of the gathered data, the grounded theory approach presumes that it is possible to discover fundamental patterns in all social life. These patterns are called 'basic social processes' (BSPs). Data collection continues until the BSP emerges. The constant comparative process is extremely rigorous in that the researcher has to reflect on categories, and must test emerging concepts and relationships many times before being able to make firm theoretical propositions.

Strauss and Corbin (1990) and Streubert and Carpenter (1999) discuss the terms associated with grounded theory, including *content comparison, memorising, theoretical sampling, bracketing, sorting, BSPs, saturation, theoretical sampling* and *theoretical sensitivity*. You can refer to these sources for further information on these terms.

Qualitative research using the grounded theory approach is becoming increasingly popular in the health sciences, as is evidenced by the growing number of articles in research journals and papers presented at research conferences.

Classical examples of grounded theory are the study on older women's experience on urinary incontinence by Dowd (1991) and the study on bereavement experience of caregivers by Jones and Martinson (1992).

Philosophical enquiry

In its broadest sense, philosophy is the process and expression of rational reflection upon experience (Hastings 1961). Russell (1945: xiii) sees philosophy as being intermediate between theology and science, and describes it thus: "All definite knowledge ... belongs to science; all dogma as to what surpasses definite knowledge belongs to theology". Hutchison (1977) distinguishes science from philosophy in terms of the range of context – whereas science deals with a limited and specific reality, or the *material* world, philosophy traditionally encompasses all-inclusive totality, or the *entire* world.

The purpose of philosophical enquiry is to perform research using intellectual analysis to clarify meaning, make values manifest, identify ethics and study the nature of knowledge (Burns & Grove 2003). Research focusing on philosophical questions is difficult to design and pursue. Many textbooks on health sciences research, or research in general, do not include this type of design, yet for the health care professionals, philosophical questions abound. For example:

- What is nursing/physiotherapy/occupational therapy?
- What are the boundaries of these sciences, or what phenomena belong to them?
- What thoughts, ideas and values are important to these sciences?
- What is the meaning and purpose of human life, if there is any meaning and purpose?
- What is the status of free will?
- What is the significance of dignity, and what does it mean to be compassionate and caring?

Many philosophical questions relating to ethics confront health care professionals, such as obligations, rights, duties, concepts of right and wrong, conscience, justice, intention and responsibility. These questions can be divided into three categories, namely, foundational studies, philosophical analysis and ethical analysis.

The philosophical researcher considers an idea or issue from every perspective through extensively exploring the literature, examining conceptual meaning, raising questions, proposing answers and suggesting the implications of those answers. The research is guided by the questions. As with other qualitative approaches, data collection occurs simultaneously with analysis, and focuses on words. The data source for most philosophical studies is written materials and verbally expressed ideas relevant to the topic of interest. The researcher often explores and debates the ideas, questions, answers and consequences with colleagues during the analysis phase.

The method in which philosophers primarily engage is *argumentation*. Regardless of whether they formulate analyses of certain concepts, draw distinctions, discuss assumptions or construct interpretations, they use arguments. Argumentation by analysis, argumentation by interpretation and argumentation by logical stricture are the specialised intellectual tools of the philosopher.

Classical examples of philosophical enquiry are Carper's (1978) study of the ways of knowing in the health sciences; Smith's (1986) idea of health; and Kayser-Jones, Davis, Wiener and Higgin's (1990) ethical analysis of an elder's treatment.

Reliability and validity in qualitative approaches

Reliability and validity with regard to research findings are of great importance in all studies. In qualitative research, however, they are often viewed with scepticism and studies are criticised for lack of rigour. But the criteria that are used to judge the rigour of qualitative studies are often those developed to judge quantitative studies. This is a mistake. Methods for establishing reliability and validity in qualitative research *differ* from those used in quantitative research. In fact, qualitative researchers tend to reject the terms 'reliability' and 'validity' in favour of 'consistency', 'dependability', 'conformability', 'auditability', 'recurrent patterning', 'credibility', 'trustworthiness' and 'transferability' (Corbin & Strauss 1990; Leininger 1991; Lincoln & Cuba 1985; Miles & Huberman 1994). In this book, we use the term 'trustworthiness'.

Reliability is concerned with the consistency, stability and repeatability of the informants' accounts, as well as the researcher's ability to collect and record information accurately (Selltiz, Wrightsman & Cook 1976). The underlying issue here, according to Miles and Huberman (1994: 278), is "whether the process of the study is consistent, reasonably stable over time and across researchers". In qualitative research this requires that a researcher using the same or comparable methods should obtain the same or comparable results every time that he/she uses the methods on the same or comparable subjects. Furthermore, the researcher must develop consistent responses, or habits, in using the method and scoring or rating its results, as well as manage factors related to participants and testing procedures to reduce measurement error.

Validity is concerned with the accuracy and truthfulness of scientific findings (Le Compte & Goetz 1982). Establishing validity requires, firstly, determining the extent to which conclusions effectively represent empirical reality and, secondly, assessing whether constructs devised by researchers represent or measure the categories of human experience that occur. In qualitative research, credibility and authenticity refer to *internal validity*. The researcher asks: 'Are the findings credible to the people I am studying as well as to my readers?' and 'Do I have an authentic portrait of what I am looking for?'.

Techniques used to achieve credibility include
- remaining in the field over a long period
- using a variety of sources in data gathering – triangulation
- peer debriefing, in which the researcher exposes him-/herself to a disinterested peer who probes the researcher's biases, explores meanings, and clarifies the bases for particular interpretations
- searching and accounting for disconfirming evidence – negative case analysis
- having the research participants review, validate and verify the researcher's interpretations and conclusions – member checking – which is done to ensure that the facts have not been misconstrued.

Authenticity can be established by context-rich and meaningful, or 'thick', descriptions (Denzin 1989).

External validity, which is defined by quantitative researchers as the degree to which the results of a study can be generalised to other settings or samples, is usually referred to as 'transferability' and/or 'fittingness' in qualitative work. The researcher asks: 'Are the conclusions of the study transferable to other contexts? Do they 'fit'?' (Lincoln & Guba 1985). He/she helps to provide a detailed database and thick description so that someone else can determine whether the findings of the study are applicable in another context or setting.

Dependability is a further criterion listed by Lincoln and Guba (1985) to establish the trustworthiness of the study. This requires an audit. The enquiry auditor – generally a peer – follows the process and procedures used by the researcher in the study and determines whether they are acceptable, that is, dependable.

Confirmability guarantees that the findings, conclusions and recommendations are supported by the data and that there is internal agreement between the investigator's interpretation and the actual evidence. This is also accomplished by incorporating an audit procedure.

Miles and Huberman (1994) give a highly detailed description of tactics and strategies for ensuring the validity and reliability of the study. If you intend conducting qualitative studies, you should read these authors' recommendations carefully.

Choice of research design

Whether it is traditional or non-traditional, quantitative or qualitative, no particular research design is considered to be more valuable than another. The best design is always the one that is most appropriate to the research problem and purpose.

Table 9.1 on the next page presents an example of how the choice of the research design varies in relation to the purpose of the study.

The example not only indicates how the choice of research design varies with the purpose, but also illustrates how at least five different research projects can evolve from one problem area – in this case obesity of teenagers – and how both quantitative and qualitative designs are appropriate, depending, of course, on the purpose.

Table 9.1 The problem of obesity in teenagers from community X: Research design and purpose

Design	Purpose of study
Descriptive, e.g. case study or survey	To describe the dietary patterns of obese teenagers in community X
Correlational	To determine the relationship between compliance with a weight reduction protocol and successful weight loss in obese teenagers residing in community X
Experimental	To compare the effectiveness of two weight-reduction protocols on the incidence of weight loss in obese teenagers resident in community X
Methodological	To develop and test the reliability and validity of an instrument to measure the influence of dietary patterns on obese teenagers
Exploratory (qualitative) (ethnographic) or Phenomenological	To explore how the obese teenagers residing in community X experience their obesity

Summary

In this chapter, we presented an overview and the distinguishing characteristics of the most common non-traditional and qualitative designs. We have explored the qualitative methods of phenomenology, ethnography, grounded theory and philosophical enquiry. Having discussed aspects pertaining to the validity and reliability of qualitative research, the chapter concluded with an example of the manner in which the choice of a research design depends on the purpose.

The intention of this chapter is simply to be an introduction. If you wish to do an in-depth study of the designs we discuss, you need to explore the texts to which we refer.

Exercises

Complete these exercises:

1 Reflect on your clinical practice and identify a research problem or question for which a qualitative research method may provide an answer. Using the characteristics of qualitative methods, describe how you might present the study.

2 Select one of the two excerpts below and complete the following activities:

   Excerpt A: A health care professional works in a paediatric oncology unit, where many of the patients are terminal. She structures an investigation to determine the grief experience of the parents of the dying children.

Excerpt B: Working in a rural clinic where many of the patients are Tsonga, a health care professional wants to investigate the cultural beliefs and customs that influence health behaviour.

a) Identify the type of qualitative research approach that would be most appropriate to use in the excerpt you selected.

b) Identify the sources of data.

c) Discuss the researcher's role in the study.

d) Briefly identify how data could be recorded and analysed.

e) Describe what could be used to add credibility to the study.

3   From a recent health sciences research journal, select an article of research in which a qualitative method is used. Identify the strategies that the researcher uses to ensure validity and reliability.

10 Sampling

LEARNING OUTCOMES

On completion of this chapter, you should be able to demonstrate your understanding of

- the purposes of sampling
- the terms 'population', 'sample', 'sampling error' and 'sampling bias'
- probability and non-probability sampling approaches
- the various techniques of probability sampling and their differences
- the various techniques of non-probability sampling and their differences
- the use of a table of random numbers to select a sample
- the factors that influence the determination of sample size
- the criteria used to evaluate the sampling section of a research report.

Introduction

Having selected and defined the research problem and decided which approach to use to investigate it, the researcher must choose, in an appropriate manner, the objects, persons and events from which the actual information needs to be drawn. Therefore, he/she needs to define the population and sample. Occasionally, the researcher may study an entire population. This is likely to occur when there are only a few persons who have the characteristics in which the researcher is interested. But as a rule, the population is too large, unwieldy and widespread to be studied directly, which raises the question of whether it is even necessary for the researcher to study the entire population. The study of each element in the population would generally take too long and be impractical and costly. The researcher thus works with samples. Furthermore, sampling may provide a more accurate picture of the phenomenon under investigation than would the measurement of all the population elements.

Research aims to optimise the use of resources in the investigation of the area of interest. Sampling is one way of doing exactly that.

Basic sampling concepts

You need to be familiar with the concepts associated with sampling in order to understand its importance in health sciences research.

Population

In the definitions used by various authors, a population is the entire group of persons or objects that is of interest to the researcher, in other words, that meets the criteria which the researcher is interested in studying (Brink & Wood 1998; Burns & Grove 2003; De Vos 2002; Polgar & Thomas 2000; Polit & Hungler 1995; Rossouw 2003). De Vos (2002: 198) furthermore describes the term as setting boundaries with regard to the elements or subjects. For instance, if a researcher studies South African health care professionals with Masters degrees, the population can be defined as all South African citizens who are health care professionals registered with a professional health council and who have obtained a degree at Masters level. Other examples of populations are all South African women with metastatic breast cancer, and all pregnant teenagers in South Africa.

But because researchers rarely have access to the entire population, the population that the researcher does have access to and actually studies usually differs in one or more aspects. This population is known as either the 'accessible population' (Burns & Grove 2003; Polit & Hungler 1995; Woods & Catanzaro 1988), or the 'study population' (Brink & Wood 1998; Struwig & Stead 2001). It is highly improbable that a researcher in Gauteng would be able to identify and find every South African woman with metastatic breast cancer. However, it may be possible for him/her to locate every South African woman with metastatic breast cancer who has been treated at South African academic hospitals in the last five years.

But even such a population may not be accessible to the researcher if, for example, entry permission is refused by an authority. In this case the researcher has to limit the accessible population by adding a characteristic to the defined population, such as restricting the setting of the study to academic hospitals in Gauteng. The researcher then plans to generalise his/her findings to this particular population, rather than the entire population. The sample of women obtained from a population treated at academic hospitals may be quite different from a sample of women treated at private hospitals, which have patients who belong to a medical aid scheme. The former group is likely to have a socio-cultural background that is different from that of the latter group. As a result, conclusions drawn from this sample would probably be invalid as regards the population in private hospitals, and hence are not generalisable to the total population.

Clearly, it is critical that the researcher carefully defines and describes the population, and specifically stipulates criteria for inclusion in it. These criteria are referred to as 'eligibility criteria', 'inclusion criteria' or 'distinguishing descriptors' (Polit & Hungler 1995). Researchers should use them as the basis for their decision of whether an individual or object would or would not be classified as a member of the population in question.

Sample

By definition, a sample is a part or fraction of a whole, or a subset of a larger set, selected by the researcher to participate in a research study. A sample thus consists of a selected group of the elements or units of analysis from a defined population. In sampling terminology the **element** is the most basic unit about which information is collected. In health sciences research, the element is typically an individual, but other entities can also form the basis of a sample or population, such as documents, blood group, events, groups of people, organisations, behaviours, or any other single measurement unit of a study (Bless & Higson-Smith 2000; Burns & Grove 2003; Polgar & Thomas 2000).

Sampling refers to the researcher's process of selecting the sample from a population in order to obtain information regarding a phenomenon in a way that represents the population of interest.

Sampling frame

The sampling frame is a comprehensive list of the sampling elements in the target population. The sample for a study is drawn from this frame. Lists of populations, such as hospital or clinic admission registers, membership lists and personnel lists, are sometimes readily available. Frequently, the researcher has to prepare a sampling frame by listing all members of the accessible population. This can be a time-consuming task, and the researcher must take care to delineate the population accurately. An inadequate sampling frame that disregards a part of the target population has been the cause of many poor research findings and results. An adequate sampling frame should therefore include *all* elements of the population under study.

Parameter and statistic

A specific measure or numerical value that relates to the population, such as age, gender, educational level, income or marital status, is called a 'population parameter'. This is the characteristic of the element or unit of analysis that is relevant to the study at hand. The corresponding measures, or numerical values or quantities, of a sample – such as 25 years of age, or 156 cm in height – are referred to as 'sample statistics'.

One of the aims of research is to describe certain characteristics of a target population. Therefore, an objective of sampling is to draw inferences about the unknown population parameters from the known sample statistics by obtaining data from the sample.

A representative sample

'Representativeness' means that the sample must be similar to the population in as many ways as possible. The former should replicate the population variables in approximately the same proportion as they occur in the latter. The demographic information that the researcher commonly looks at includes educational level, gender, ethnicity, age and income level, as these tend to influence the study variables. For example, if age and educational level are variables, or population parameters, relevant to the study, then a representative sample will have closely similar proportions, or representativeness, of the same age groups and levels of education as the target population.

Representativeness is extremely important when the researcher wants to generalise from the sample to the target population by drawing conclusions about the population from which the sample came.

Sampling error

Sampling error is the difference between a sample statistic and a population parameter. A large sampling error indicates that the sample is failing to provide a precise picture of the population; that is, it is not representative. Sampling error is not under the researcher's control; it is caused by chance variations that may occur when a sample is chosen to represent the population. It is difficult for the researcher to provide statistics exactly equal to the population parameters that they are to estimate. Sampling error is more likely to occur if the population or sample size is relatively small. The larger the sample and the more homogeneous the population, the smaller the sampling error. When the researcher uses careful probability sampling, he/she can estimate the degree of error statistically.

Sampling error may occur owing to the following:

- The **chance factor** – one element and not another has been included by chance. These errors can be calculated statistically and can never be completely eliminated.
- **Bias in selection** – primarily resulting from incorrect technique. These biases are often avoidable, and may or may not be deliberate.
- **Non-response error** – when, for an unknown reason, an element does not respond to the measurement instrument. Because these elements are now excluded from the sample, the constitution of the sample, and thus the representativeness, changes.

Sampling bias

Sampling bias is caused by the researcher. It occurs when samples are not carefully selected. Sources of sampling bias can be the time of day or year when the data were collected, the place in which they were gathered, the language used, the extent to which personal views colour the data, the use of an incomplete or incorrect sampling frame, or the researcher being guided by preference in the selection of research subject.

Sampling approaches

There are two basic sampling approaches – probability or random sampling and non-probability sampling – which we will now discuss along with their related techniques.

Probability or random sampling

Here, the sample is much more likely to be representative of the population and to reflect its variations. It implies that all elements in the population have an equal chance of being included in the sample. Probability sampling also permits the researcher to estimate the sampling error, reduces bias in the sample or sampling, and makes it possible for the researcher to use inferential statistics correctly. When the researcher's primary concern in selecting a sample is to obtain findings that can be generalised to the population, a probability sample would be the sample of choice.

To obtain a probability sample, the researcher must know *every* element in the population. There must be an available listing of all members of the population, and the sample must be randomly selected from the list. The list is the single most important criterion in determining whether probability sampling is possible for a given study. If it is possible, then one of the common techniques of probability samples may be used. These include *simple random sampling, stratified random sampling, systematic random sampling* and *cluster sampling*.

Techniques or types of probability or random sampling

The selection of an element or unit from a population is called 'random' when each element or unit has the same chance, likelihood or probability of being chosen for the sample. The probability samples we describe below all use the process of random selection.

Simple random sampling

Simple random samples are drawn using the basic probability sampling technique. Subjects or elements are drawn in a random way from the sampling frame. Each of the elements in the frame is listed separately and therefore has an equal chance of being included in the sample.

The main features of a simple random sample are that

- it involves a one-stage selection process
- each subject or object has an equal and independent chance of being drawn
- the study or accessible population can be identified and listed.

Using this technique, the researcher needs to follow these steps:

1 Define the population.
2 Create a sample frame.
3 Calculate the sample size.
4 Assign a consecutive identification number to each element in the sample frame.
5 Select a technique to randomly sample the subjects.

There are various techniques of selecting randomly. The most common entail

- placing the numbers or names in a bowl or hat and drawing them out one at a time, otherwise known as the 'fishbowl technique'
- using a table of random numbers
- using a computer-generated selection of random numbers.

When using the fishbowl technique, the researcher must follow these steps:

1 Write each name or number from the sampling frame, or the list, on a separate slip of paper. For example, if the defined study population consists of all medical doctors in hospital X and there are 100 on the personnel list, the researcher writes out 100 slips.
2 Put the slips into the bowl, hat or other suitable container.
3 Draw a slip, note the name or number, replace the slip, shake the bowl and select

a second, and a third, and so on, until there is the required number according to the sample size which the researcher calculated. Note that each slip must be replaced after each selection. This ensures that each participant has an equal and independent chance of being selected each time. When this approach is used, each of the 100 names has a 1-in-100 chance of being selected each time. This is called 'random sampling with replacement'. If in this case a participant is selected twice, the researcher should ignore the duplicate and repeat the process until he/she has the required sample. Where 20 names have been selected without returning the slip to the bowl, there would be a 1-in-80 chance of selection. This is called 'random sampling without replacement'.

To use a table of random numbers, the researcher can follow this procedure:

1 Find a table of random numbers, which is available in most statistical books. Tables 10.1 and 10.2 present an excerpt from such a table. The table is mathematically prepared so that numbers are written in a random manner in rows or columns. Alternatively, the researcher can generate a table of random numbers by computer. This is effective even when large populations are involved.
2 Select a starting point by pointing to a place on the table without looking at it.
3 Beginning with the number selected, choose a direction – that is, horizontal, vertical or diagonal – and continue in a systematic fashion to select the desired number of participants.
4 If a number occurs in a row or column that is not represented in the population, exclude the number and move to the next one.

Table 10.1 Table of random numbers

46	85	04	23	26
69	24	89	34	60
14	01	33	17	92
56	30	38	73	15
81	30	44	85	85

Source: Adapted from Polit and Hungler (1991: 156)

Table 10.2 Sample selected

The researcher needs ten subjects randomly selected from a population of individuals numbered from 1 to 80 and arbitrarily begins

Subjects selected are numbers

33	38	44	23	34	17
73	26	60	15		

Source: Adapted from Polit and Hungler (1991: 156)

In the example above, the population consists of 80 individuals, which implies that two-digit numbers have to be selected. The arbitrary starting point is 33. The researcher moves down the column and then continues down the next two columns, until he/she has selected 10 numbers. He/she has to exclude two numbers that are not represented in the population numbers – 85 and 92.

In another example, out of a population of 400 the researcher must randomly select 40 units. As 400 consists of three digits, the researcher has to select any three adjacent digits and, reading row- or column-wise, write down 40 numbers under the value of 400. Using the random numbers in the above figure, starting in the top column of the top row, and moving along the top row, the first number is 468, the second one is 504. Both these must be excluded as they are not represented in the population numbers. The first number that is represented in the population is 232.

A third way of producing a simple random sample also requires that each individual be numbered. Instead of a table of random numbers, a computer-generated set of numbers is used. Commonly, more numbers are generated than are expected to constitute the sample because there may be duplications, which will have to be ignored.

Systematic or interval sampling

Systematic sampling involves selecting elements at equal intervals, such as every fifth, eighth or twentieth element. This technique is based on the supposition that cases are not added to the list in a systematic way that coincides with the sampling system. If a list of elements or cases is available, systematic sampling is easy and convenient. Moreover, it is often used in clinical practice where, for instance, patients' temperature and blood pressure is measured every hour.

In systematic sampling, the researcher should follow this procedure:

1 Obtain a list of the total population (N). The elements of this list must be listed randomly. If placed in a specific order, for example alphabetically, or in hierarchical order or males followed by females, bias may occur in that the sample selection may not be truly representative of the population.
2 Determine the sample size (n).
3 Determine the sampling interval (K) by dividing the size of the population by the size of the sample.

$$\text{sampling interval (K)} = \frac{\text{size of population}}{\text{size of the sample}} = \frac{N}{n}$$

4 Choose a random starting point – the best way is through a table of random numbers.
5 Select the other elements or units based on the sampling interval. For example, if the population is 400 and the sample size is 80, the sampling interval is 5 (400 ÷ 80). A number between 1 and 400 is randomly selected as the starting number. Imagining that the first randomly selected number is 12, the next four subjects will be 17, 22, 27 and 32.

When careful attention is paid to obtaining an unbiased listing of the population elements, and the first element is randomly selected, systematic sampling is classified as probability sampling. If either of the criteria is not met, non-probability sampling occurs.

Stratified random sampling

In stratified random sampling, the population is divided into subgroups or strata according to a variable or variables of importance to the study, so that each element of the population belongs to one and only one stratum. Then, within each stratum, random sampling is performed, using either the simple or systematic (interval) sampling technique. There are various characteristics of population that may call for the use of stratified sampling. Subject characteristics such as age, gender, educational level and income are examples of variables that might be used as criteria for dividing populations into subgroups. For hospitals, the strata may be such characteristics as size, state or private, or the number of beds.

For example, the researcher has chosen size as the number of beds in a hospital, and is seeking a 50% sample of this group of hospitals. Table 10.3 provides the relevant random sample.

Table 10.3 Example of a random sample stratified according to size

Size	No of hospitals	Proportional sample (50%)
>1 000	6	3
500–999	8	4
200–499	16	8
<200	20	10
	50	25

In this illustration, the hospitals are listed in groups according to size. Using a table of random numbers, the researcher draws a 50% sample from each of the groups. The resulting sample consists of 25 hospitals, with all sizes represented in the same proportion that they were in the population. The researcher has therefore selected a proportionate stratified random sample. All the segments are proportionately represented, which is particularly important when key segments in the population occur in low proportions. Furthermore, the exact representativeness of the sample is known, which has important statistical value.

Disproportionate stratified sampling occurs when the number of elements in each stratum is not proportionate to the number in the population. In the above example, instead of selecting a 50% sample from each stratum, the researcher could have selected five hospitals from each group.

The advantage of stratified random sampling is that it provides for the representation of a particular segment of the population. The disadvantages are that it requires extensive knowledge of the population in order for it to be stratified, a complete list of the study population is needed, it can be costly and it can quickly become highly complex.

Cluster random sampling

In large-scale studies, where the population is geographically widespread, sampling procedures can be difficult and time-consuming. In addition, it may be difficult or even impossible for the researcher to obtain a total listing of some populations. In this case, cluster sampling may be appropriate.

Cluster sampling takes place in stages. The researcher begins with the largest, most inclusive sampling unit, and progresses to the next most inclusive sampling unit until he/she reaches the final stage, which is the selection of the elements or participants in the study. For example, a researcher who wishes to study cancer patients across the country may use regions in South Africa as the largest unit – that is, the nine provinces in the country – and then randomly select a sample from the provinces. Next, he/she identifies the hospitals which admit and treat cancer patients in each of the provinces making up the sample. He/she selects a sample of the hospitals, probably by stratified sampling. The final selection is a sample of cancer patients from the selected sample of hospitals. In summary, the clusters considered in this example are provinces, hospitals and, finally, patients. The specification of each cluster constitutes a stage, and each stage is characterised by a random sample.

The main advantage of cluster sampling is that it is considerably more economical in terms of time and costs than other techniques of probability sampling, particularly when the population is large and geographically dispersed.

However, there are two major disadvantages:

1 More sampling errors tend to occur than with simple random or stratified random sampling, especially in the first stage, which is aggravated in the following stages.
2 The appropriate handling of the statistical data from cluster samples is extremely complex.

Non-probability sampling

This type of sampling may or may not accurately represent the population. It is usually more convenient and economical, and allows the study of populations when they are not amenable to probability sampling, or when the researcher is unable to locate the entire population. Where access to the subjects or elements is limited, the representativeness of the sample also cannot be determined, because it will be impossible for the researcher to specify whether each element has an equal chance of being included in the sample.

Non-probability sampling requires the researcher to judge and select those subjects who know the most about the phenomenon, and who are able to articulate and explain nuances to him/her. The non-probability sampling plan is constructed from an objective judgement of a likely starting point, and the direction that the sampling takes will be a decision made by the researcher as the study progresses (Field & Morse 1985). The major techniques of non-probability samples include *purposive or theoretical samples, convenience samples, quota samples* and *special technique samples* such as *snowball or network samples.*

This type of sampling places a much greater burden of judgement on the researcher. The major disadvantages are that it does not contribute to generalisation, that the extent of sampling error cannot be estimated and that bias may be present. Nevertheless, this approach is defensible in many instances. For example, the researcher may not be concerned with the typical experience of the population and therefore is not interested in generalisability. Instead, he/she may be more concerned with understanding the experience of special segments of the population, or interested in studying rare or unpredictable phenomena.

The quality of the data obtained from non-probability samples has the potential to be high if the researchers are dealing with willing and able subjects. The significance of the results has the same potential, depending on the logical and theoretical direction that the researcher can impose on the sampling process. Taking care in the selection of the sample, conservatively interpreting the results, and replicating the study with new samples, the researcher may find that non-probability samples work well.

In many situations, especially in studies of a clinical nature, the researcher may have to use a non-probability approach if he/she does not wish to abandon the project altogether. Even uncompromising research consultants would hesitate to advocate the total abandonment of a researcher's ideas in the absence of a random sample.

Techniques or types of non-probability sampling

In non-probability sampling, the sampling elements are chosen from the population by non-random methods.

Convenience sampling

Convenience sampling is also referred to as 'accidental' or 'availability sampling', and it involves the choice of readily available subjects or objects for the study. Although this technique is used frequently it is considered a poor type of sampling because it provides little opportunity to control bias. Elements are included in the sample because they happen to be in the right place at the right time. The researcher may choose, for example, the first 20 patients arriving at an antenatal clinic for an interview, or the patients available in a specific ward on a certain day; or a lecturer may use students in his/her class. Obviously, this can introduce certain biases, as some elements may be over-represented or under-represented. Generalisation based on such samples is extremely risky, although the samples so chosen are convenient for researchers in terms of time and costs. While this type of sampling is used in studies where probability sampling is not possible, it should be used only when samples are unobtainable by other means, especially in quantitative studies.

Quota sampling

This sampling technique could be considered the non-probability equivalent of stratified sampling. The purpose is to draw a sample that has the same proportions or characteristics as the entire population. However, instead of relying on random choice, the sampling procedure relies on convenience choice. The aim of quota sampling is to replicate the proportions of subgroups or strata present in the population.

The researcher first determines which strata are to be studied. Common strata are age groups, gender, race, geographic locations and socio-economic groups. The researcher then determines a quota, or number of participants, needed for each stratum. The quota may be determined proportionately or disproportionately. For a proportionate quota sample, the researcher must obtain information on the composition of the population. If the population consists of 60% women, the sample should also consist of 60% women. The ratio is thus the same.

For example, the population under study is estimated to consist of 40% men and 60% women. Twenty-five per cent of the men are older than 40 and 15% are between 20 and 40 years of age. Of the 60% women, 30% are in each of these age groups. If the researcher intends to draw a sample of 200, he/she interviews people in each stratum 'as they come', that is, using convenience sampling, until he/she has gathered 80 men (40% of 200), of whom 50 are older than 40 and 30 are between 20 and 40 years of age. The female subsample consists of 120 women, 60 in each age category. Disproportionate sampling would occur, for example, if the researcher decided to use 50% males and 50% females and 25% from each of the age groups.

Purposive/theoretical/judgemental sampling

Purposive sampling is sometimes also called 'judgemental' or 'theoretical sampling' (Brink & Wood 1998; Glaser & Strauss 1967). It is another type of non-probability sampling. Thus this technique is based on the judgement of the researcher regarding subjects or objects that are typical or representative of the study phenomenon, or who are especially knowledgeable about the question at hand. Alternatively, the researcher may wish to interview individuals who reflect different ends of the range of a particular characteristic. A simple example is a comparison between patients who display a low pain threshold and those who experience a high pain threshold. In a more complex example, a researcher who wants to investigate attitudes towards death in HIV-positive individuals may select subjects who have no symptoms and those who have active disease and are considered terminal. It can also be used when specific cases are needed for deep analysis.

This type of sampling is commonly seen in qualitative research. As the qualitative researcher using this method does not know in advance how many subjects are needed, he/she samples continuously until data saturation occurs. Data saturation is the point at which new data no longer emerge during the data-collection process.

'Theoretical sampling' is the term applied to a more elaborate process used in conjunction with the analysis of data in grounded theory. As the analysis reveals the relationships between the elements of the emerging theory, new sample subjects are sought to clarify, extend and refute the findings (Brink & Wood 1998: 320).

The advantage of purposive sampling is that it allows the researcher to select the sample based on knowledge of the phenomena being studied. The disadvantages are the potential for sampling bias, the use of a sample that does not represent the population, and the limited generalisability of the results.

Snowball sampling

Snowball sampling involves the assistance of study subjects in obtaining other potential subjects, especially where it is difficult for the researcher to gain access to the population. This type of sampling consists of different stages. Firstly, the researcher identifies a few people who have the required characteristics. They then help him/her to identify more people, who also possess the desired characteristics and who are included in the next stage. The process continues until the researcher is satisfied that the sample is sufficiently large. For example, the researcher wants to determine how to help people to stop smoking. He/she may know or hear of someone who has been successful in refraining from smoking for several years. This person is contacted and asked if he/she knows others who have also been successful. This type of networking is particularly helpful in finding people who are reluctant to make their identity known.

Choice of sample

The choice of the sample is also closely related to the study design. For example, in the case of a researcher studying an area in which little knowledge has accumulated, he/she would select a level 1 question and a qualitative design. A probability sample would not be suitable in this instance. If, however, he/she seeks to test hypotheses, a non-probability sample would be unsuitable. The suitability of a particular type of sampling for a particular type of design could be controversial when there is an overlap between possible types of design. The relationships depicted in Table 10.4, however, serve as useful guidelines for novice researchers.

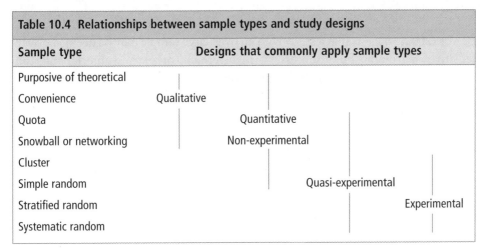

Table 10.4 Relationships between sample types and study designs

Sample type	Designs that commonly apply sample types
Purposive of theoretical	
Convenience	Qualitative
Quota	Quantitative
Snowball or networking	Non-experimental
Cluster	
Simple random	Quasi-experimental
Stratified random	Experimental
Systematic random	

Source: Adapted from Roberts and Burke (1989: 217)

Sample size

Selecting the appropriate sample size and obtaining the required size are problems that face every researcher. Many give little thought to sample size, and instead work on preconceived ideas, regardless of the purpose of the study and the research design, and choose the most convenient number. Such samples can give misleading results and should be viewed with scepticism. As is true of much of the research process, there are no hard and fast rules that can be applied to the determination of sample size; however, the researcher must consider both scientific and pragmatic factors influencing the sample size when he/she decides on the number of subjects to be included in the study. These factors vary with the purpose, design and type of sample used. Therefore, sample size cannot be transferred from one study to another, but must be calculated anew for each research problem.

It is often stated that the larger the sample, the better it is. While a large sample is often an advantage in quantitative studies, evidence exists that this holds true only up to a point and is not applicable to qualitative studies. After a certain size is reached, increasing the size does not improve the matter significantly. Giovanetti (1981) states that as the population increases in size, the sample size required for precision in estimation remains constant, and that the absolute size of the sample is more important than the sample size relative to population size. Furthermore, with regard to a probability sample and the precision of how closely the sample value relates to the population value, she suggests that 'equal precision' is found in the following samples:

■ When the population is 2 000 and the sample is 200, (10% of the population).
■ When the population is 100 000 and the sample is 200, (2% of the population) (Giovanetti 1981).

De Vos (2002) suggests that a study with an over-large sample may be deemed overly sensitive. Through the unnecessary involvement of extra subjects and the correspondingly increased costs, it can become unethical. Similarly, a study with a sample that is too small will be unable to detect clinically important effects and may thus be scientifically useless, and hence unethical in its use of subjects and other resources. In addition, a large sample is no guarantee of accuracy – a large sample with a poor design can inflate error and bias.

When using probability sampling in quantitative studies, the researcher can calculate the exact number of subjects needed according to how much sampling error he/she is willing to accept. Ader and Mellenbergh (1999), Cohen (1977), and Polgar and Thomas (2000) provide formulae for calculating the effect of size, and tables for many types of statistical tests that show the required sample size.

As we mention above, the proposition that a larger sample is better does not apply in qualitative studies, where the type of sample is usually purposive. Too many subjects would cloud the issues and increase the complexity of the analysis process. For these types of studies, the sample size is adequate when the meanings are clear and data are fully explored (Breakwell, Hammond & Fife-Schaw 2000; Field & Morse 1985; Polit & Hungler 1995). The trend, however, indicates a shift away from samples that are too small to numbers of 20 or even 30 in qualitative studies. Sample sizes smaller than this imply that the meanings will be idiosyncratic, and they make it difficult for the researcher to observe the identity of the subjects. Nevertheless, it is important that data saturation is reached.

Besides the nature of the design and the degree of precision required, several other factors should be considered in the determination of the sample size.

These include the following:

■ **Precision of the data-collection instrument.** In general, a study that uses a crude measure will have to sample more subjects to obtain a reasonable estimate of a population parameter than is the case when the data-collection instrument is more precise. The less precise the tool, the larger the sample needed.
■ **Heterogeneity of the population.** As the number of demographic variables increases, so must the sample size. Most researchers agree that there should be at least 10 subjects for each variable in the sample, with 20 to 30 per variable preferred (Polit & Hungler 1995).

■ **Incidence of the type of subject in the population.** In cases where the incidence of the study phenomenon is rare, larger numbers of subjects are required for survey than in the case of a common phenomenon. The statistical analyses also impose certain requirements regarding sample size.

Table 10.5 Factors influencing the choice of a sample size	
Factor	**Things to remember and consider**
Accuracy needed	As the sample increases (to a point), the accuracy increases
Size of population	As the size of population increases, a progressively smaller proportion of subjects can be selected Survey designs frequently require large numbers of subjects
Nature of research design	Qualitative studies are conducted with fewer subjects
Type of research	Preferably a minimum of 30 subjects is needed per variable or phenomenon
Heterogeneity	As the number of variables increases, the sample size must grow (more subjects are needed)
Methods of data collection	If methods are not precise, a larger sample is required
Research hypothesis	When slight differences are expected, a larger sample is required
Statistical analyses to be used	Sample size can be written as the value of the indicators
Financial resources	Must be in relation to availability of resources
Attrition rate	Often expected, may influence sample size

Table 10.5 summarises the factors that the researcher must consider when choosing a sample size.

Sampling is an integral part of the research process, and should not be considered in isolation. When planning samples, the researcher should consider the sample in relation to purpose and design, as well as practical reality. This is beneficial because it reduces the time and costs that the researcher needs to complete the study.

Sample adequacy

It is important that both the researcher and the research consumer evaluate the adequacy of the sample in a research study. Several aspects of the sampling procedure must be systematically evaluated. A checklist for the evaluation is presented in Table 10.6 on the next page.

Table 10.6 Evaluation checklist	
1	Are the target population, accessible population and sample described?
2	Was a probability or non-probability sampling method used?
3	Is the specific sampling method or technique named and described?
4	Does the type of sample fit with the type of design?
5	Does the type of sample fit with the purpose of the study?
6	If a non-probability sampling approach is used, how is representativeness accounted for in the sample?
7	Is a methodological or theoretical rationale for the sample size clearly explained?
8	Is the sample size similar to those in similar studies?
9	For qualitative studies, do there seem to be enough subjects to describe the phenomenon, but not so many as to cloud the issues?
10	For studies with a probability sample, was a power analysis done?
11	Are inclusion or eligibility criteria listed?
12	Is any attrition of subjects (subject drop-out) clearly described?
13	Are inclusion or eligibility criteria listed?
14	Are these biases reflected in the interpretation of the results section of the report?
15	Have sources of sampling error been controlled or minimised?
16	Is enough information given so that another researcher would be able to replicate the sampling procedures?

Summary

In this chapter, we paid attention to the various aspects of sampling, and explained the basic sampling concepts. We described the two major approaches to sampling, as well as the common techniques or types. The chapter closed by exploring sample size and giving guidelines for evaluating the adequacy of a sample.

Exercises

Complete these exercises:

1 What is the rationale behind the use of samples? Should samples be used only when a complete list of a population is unavailable? Give reasons for your answer.

2 As a researcher, you would like to study the effects of music on mentally disturbed persons. In this regard, answer these questions:
   a) What would be your target population?
   b) What would be your accessible population?
   c) What are your inclusion or eligibility criteria?

3 Using the table of random numbers we provide in Table 10.1, draw a sample of five units out of a population of 270.

4 Select an article from a research journal. Evaluate the sampling section of the research report.

11 Data collection

LEARNING OUTCOMES

On completion of this chapter, you should be able to demonstrate your understanding of

- the questions that guide the data-collection process
- the major data-collection methods
- factors that affect the selection or development of data-collection methods in quantitative research
- the advantages and disadvantages of interviews and questionnaires
- two methods of sampling observations
- the construction of a questionnaire
- the differences between the three levels of structure that can be used in interviews
- the similarities and contrasts between the various types of data-collection techniques.

Introduction

In this chapter, we focus on data-collection procedures and techniques, which are planned as part of the research design. The process of data collection is of critical importance to the success of a study. Without high quality data-collection techniques, the accuracy of the research conclusions is easily challenged. It is therefore essential that the researcher is familiar with the various data-collection techniques, including their advantages and disadvantages, so that he/she can select the most suitable technique for the study purpose, the setting and the proposed study population.

Data-collection process

When planning the process of data collection, the researcher is guided by five important questions:

1 What?
2 How?
3 Who?
4 Where?
5 When?

We will now explore each of these.

What data will be collected?

The researcher must carefully consider exactly what type of information is needed to answer the research question. For example, does the question call for knowledge, or attitudes or behaviours? If the researcher is concerned with the way crisis situations affect students, the *what* of data collection becomes students' behaviours or responses in crises. The researchers must also consider if he/she is going to quantify the data or analyse it qualitatively. In the former case, a decision must be made regarding the level of measurement or measurement scale to be used.

Nominal scales

Nominal scales are used when persons, events or other phenomena are separated into mutually exclusive categories, for example married or single, divorced or widowed, dead or alive. Even feelings can be classified using nominal scales – a person can be happy or sad, angry or calm, and so on.

Ordinal scales

Ordinal scales are used for variables that can be categorised and rank ordered or assessed incrementally. For example, the feelings of a person are classified not only as happy or sad, but also more specifically as extremely happy, happy, indifferent, unhappy or extremely unhappy, thus enabling the comparison between *degrees* of a person's happiness. Other examples of ordinal scales are 1 plus, 2 plus, 3 plus pitting oedema; and slight, moderate or intense pain. In the latter case, it would be appropriate for the researcher to conclude that intense pain is greater than moderate pain. However, he/she cannot determine the exact quantity of pain difference between moderate and intense, as pain cannot be measured directly.

Interval scales

Variables within the interval scale of measurement are assigned real numbers that are categorised and ordered with equal measurement between each category. The categories in interval data are the actual numbers on a scale, like those on a thermometer. If body temperature is being measured, a reading of 36,2 °C could be one category, while 37,0 °C is another category and 37,8 °C constitutes a third category. The researcher would be correct in saying that there is a difference of 0,8 °C between the first and second categories, as well as between the second and third categories; that is, there are equal intervals. Similarly, if the researcher undertakes a study in which a psychological test is used, the scores on the test would represent interval data. Let us imagine that 200 people did the test; 90 obtained scores between 40 and 49, 30 between 50 and 59, 60 between 60 and 69, and 20 between 70 and 79. These scores are categorised into interval classes; they are ranked and the measurements between each class are equal.

Ratio scales

Ratio level of measurement includes data that can be categorised and ranked. The distance between ranks can be specified and a true or natural zero point can be identified. The amount of money in your bank account, for example, could be considered ratio data because it is possible for it to be zero. In the case of the number of pain medication requests made by two groups of patients, for example, it is possible that some subjects in one group do not ask for pain medication. This type of data would be considered ratio data. Other obvious ratio scales include time, length and weight.

We further discuss these four measurement scales in Chapter 13. If the researcher designs a qualitative study, he/she is not concerned with measurement scales and instead collects data in the narrative form. The type of data that is needed also governs the *how, who, where* and *when* of the data-collection process. The answers to these questions are interrelated.

How will the data be collected?

The researcher must use a research instrument to gather the data. The type of instrument can vary from a checklist to a self-report questionnaire to a highly sophisticated physiological measure. The choice of instrument is a major decision that should be made only after careful consideration of the alternatives.

Who will collect the data?

If the researcher is going to collect all of the data, this question is easy to answer. Frequently, however, there are teams of researchers collecting data, and at times people outside the research team may be used in this phase. Data collectors can be paid for their services. Whenever more than one person is involved, it is necessary to ensure that the data are being gathered in the same manner. The data collectors need training, and the reliability of the collected data needs to be checked.

Where will the data be collected?

The setting for data collection must be carefully determined. It could take place, for example, in a carefully controlled laboratory, a classroom, a ward, a clinic, a home, a community centre, within a specific region, and so on.

When will the data be collected?

The researcher must decide exactly when the data is to be collected, as well as how long the process will last. Frequently, the only way to answer this question is by conducting a trial run or pilot study.

Data-collection techniques

There are various data-collection techniques. The ones used most frequently by health care professionals are observation, self-report and physiological methods. We will now provide an overview of these as well as other, less commonly used techniques.

Observation

Observation is a technique for collecting *descriptive* data on behaviour, events and situations. It is extremely useful in health care sciences studies because it allows the researcher to observe behaviour as it occurs. To be considered scientific, observation must be made under precisely defined conditions in a systematic and objective manner and with careful record-keeping. All observations must be checked and controlled. These criteria transform the simple act of observing the world into the purposeful act of collecting research data through observation.

Observations may be structured or unstructured. **Structured observations** entail specifying in advance precisely the behaviours or events that are to be observed and how they will be recorded, and preparing forms for record-keeping such as checklists, categorisation systems and rating scales. Structured observation is the method most commonly used in quantitative studies, where the researcher or trained observer simply observes and records certain aspects of the subjects' behaviour. Examples are health care professionals' willingness to interact with and listen to patients, and children's reactions to the removal of a plaster cast from one of their legs or arms. In the latter case, the behaviours to be observed may be distress, cooperation and a need for information. The researcher could prepare a rating scale that provides a score on these behaviours. He/she then records on the scale what he/she observes. Other examples are the interaction between a mother and her newborn baby, verbal communication behaviours when handing over the patient report, and a patient's eating habits. Structured observation requires knowledge on the part of the researcher of the expected range of behaviours in a given situation. When developing a checklist, for instance, the researcher must list *all* expected behaviours related to the variable being measured.

Unstructured observation involves the collection of descriptive information that is analysed qualitatively rather than quantitatively. In unstructured observations, the researcher attempts to describe events or behaviours as they occur, with no preconceived ideas of what he/she will see. An unstructured observation method may be used, for example, to describe the behaviour of a nurse immediately following the death of one of her patients. It would involve a complete description of everything the nurse says and does at this time. The most common forms of record-keeping in unstructured observation studies are logs and field notes. A log is a daily record of events and conversations that have taken place. Field notes may include the daily log, but tend to encompass more than a simple list of occurrences.

Observations can also be categorised according to the degree of *researcher involvement*. Spradley (1980) outlines five types of participation, ranging from non-participation, where there is no involvement with the research subjects, to complete participation, where there is total involvement with the subjects and environment. Table 11.1 on the next page illustrates the degrees of involvement.

Timing of observations

Since it is usually impossible for the researcher to observe behaviours for extended periods of time owing to fatigue and, in some cases, boredom, it is necessary for him/her to plan when and how to make the observations. Following are examples of nurse-patient interaction. The two primary methods are time sampling and event sampling. **Time sampling** involves observations of events during certain specified times. For example, to observe nurse–patient interaction, several 15-minute periods during an 8-hour shift would provide a good sample of interactions. The periods can be either randomly selected or predetermined according to the daily routine of the ward.

Event sampling involves observation of an entire event. For example, if a researcher is interested in determining nurse–patient interaction during admission to a hospital, event sampling would be appropriate because the researcher would observe the whole admission procedure. In this case, the researcher must either have some knowledge concerning the occurrence of events or be in a position to wait for their occurrence.

Table 11.1 Degrees of researcher involvement in observation research

Involvement	Participation	Example
High	Complete	Here the researcher joins the group under investigation as one of its mentors, sharing in all activities, e.g. working on a ward as a nurse, doing active patient care, while studying nurse–patient interaction. Thus, the researcher participates actively without the knowledge or consent of the participants
	Active	Similar to above, but the researcher, though considerably involved with the activities in the group, participates as researcher and not as one of the group. The researcher thus discloses his/her identity and purpose to other participants
	Moderate	The researcher interacts with members of the group while studying the activities, e.g. nurse–patient interaction, but is less involved with the actual activities
Low	Passive	The researcher studies the activities, e.g. nurse–patient interaction, merely as an observer, with little interaction or involvement with the group
None	Non-participant	The researcher studies the activities, e.g. nurse–patient interaction, in situations removed from the subjects' immediate environment – for example, from a viewing gallery or one-way mirror – no interaction or involvement, only direct observation

Source: Adapted from Spradley (1980)

Advantages and disadvantages of observation

Scientific observation has several advantages as a data-collection method. There are many health care problems that are better suited to an observational approach than to questionnaires or interviews, as what people say that they do is often not what they actually do. Examples of situations in which observation is suitable are the manifestation of pre-operative signs of anxiety, displays of aggression or hostility. In addition, no other data-collection method can match the depth and variety of information that can be collected through observational techniques. These techniques are also fairly flexible and can be used in both experimental and non-experimental designs, and in laboratory and field studies.

However, observation also has disadvantages. There are problems concerning the reactions of the observed when they are aware that they are being observed. Ethical problems can arise if the researcher does not obtain consent. The data obtained through observation are vulnerable to bias and distortion. Emotions, prejudices and values can all influence the way that behaviours and events are observed. And finally, observation is time-consuming and can be extremely costly, particularly when the observers have to be trained.

Guidelines for critiquing observational methods

The following aspects should be considered when observation has been used:

- Is observation an appropriate approach to obtain the necessary information to answer the research question?
- What or who has to be observed?
- Was a structured or unstructured approach used and to what extent was the researcher involved?
- Where did the observations actually take place?
- How were data recorded?
- What steps were taken to minimise observer bias?

Self-report techniques

When the researcher's objective is to find out what people believe, think or know, the easiest and most effective method is to direct the questions to the person concerned. As well as to gather factual information about the subjects, the purpose of questions is to find out their thoughts, perceptions, attitudes, beliefs, feelings, motives, plans, experiences, knowledge levels and memories. As subjects must answer the questions about the study variable directly, these techniques are known as self-report techniques. Logically, self-report instruments include questionnaires, scales and interviews.

The type of self-report instrument chosen depends on the research objectives and the sample. Verbal techniques such as interviews, and written techniques such as questionnaires and scales, have differing strengths and weaknesses. The researcher needs to take these aspects into account when choosing the instrument. Table 11.2 on the next page presents the advantages or strengths and disadvantages or weaknesses of questionnaires and interviews.

Questionnaires

In the questionnaire process, the respondent, who is the unit of analysis, writes down his/her answers in response to questions printed in a document. A well-designed questionnaire is easy for the respondent to address if he/she is literate. It is also easy for the researcher to administer and score. Yet such a questionnaire is difficult to develop. Each aspect, from the questions themselves to the colour of the paper used, can influence the respondents' replies. Therefore, the researcher must pay careful attention to the development or construction of the questionnaire.

Table 11.2 Strengths and weaknesses of interviews and questionnaires	
Interview	Questionnaire
Strengths	
1 The subject need not be able to read or write	1 Questionnaires are a quick way of obtaining data from a large group of people
2 Responses can be obtained from a wide range of subjects (almost all segments of the population)	2 Questionnaires are less expensive in terms of time and money
3 Responses and retention role is high	3 Questionnaires are one of the easiest research instruments to test for reliability and validity
4 Non-verbal behaviour and mannerisms can be observed	4 Subjects feel a greater sense of anonymity and are more likely to provide honest answers
5 Questions may be clarified if they are misunderstood	5 The format is standard for all subjects and is not dependent on mood of interviewer
6 In-depth responses can be obtained	
Weaknesses	
1 Training programmes are needed for interviewers	1 Mailing of questionnaires may be expensive
2 Interviews are time-consuming and expensive	2 Response rate may be low
3 Arrangements for interviews may be difficult to make	3 Respondents may provide socially acceptable answers
4 Subjects may provide socially acceptable responses	4 Respondents may fail to answer some of the items
5 Subjects may be anxious because answers are being recorded	5 There is no opportunity to clarify any items that may be misunderstood by subjects
6 Subjects may be influenced by interviewer characteristics	6 Subjects must be literate
7 Interviewers may misinterpret non-verbal behaviour	7 The subjects who respond may not be representative of the population

A well-designed questionnaire should
- meet the objectives of the enquiry
- demonstrate a fit between its contents and the research problem, and objectives
- obtain the most complete and accurate information possible, and do so within reasonable limits of time and resources.

When developing a questionnaire, as the researcher you must bear in mind these important points:

1 List the specific research issues to be investigated by the questionnaire. Clearly specified goals and objectives, or research questions and/or unambiguous hypotheses, are significant precursors to asking the right question.

2 Ensure that you have a thorough understanding of the relevant literature.

3 Analyse what kind of information is needed to study the research questions. Here, you can be aided by the use of a specification matrix of the various content areas in which questions covering specific situations are needed. Having identified the areas, you must decide what proportion of questioning time to allocate to each aspect of the content. For example, if you are interested in knowledge of and attitudes towards the use of restraints with regard to hospitalised geriatric patients, the specification matrix may resemble that provided in Figure 11.1. This matrix directs you to develop 10 questions for each cell for a total questionnaire length of 40 questions. This relatively simple matrix shows that the researcher considers all the elements to be equally important.

	Chemical restraints	Mechanical restraints
Knowledge	10	10
Attitudes	10	10

Figure 11.1 An example of a specification matrix

4 Formulate the specific questions and test each one for precision of expression, relevance, objectivity, suitability and the probability of reception and return (Leedy 1993).

We will now explore the various aspects of questionnaire formulation. In order to obtain a certain type of answer, the researcher needs to carefully consider the **construction** of the questions. He/she may seek a long, detailed answer that reflects the individuality of the respondents, or a short answer selected from given categories. In other words, the researcher has to choose between using unstructured, open-ended questions or structured, closed-ended questions. The former allow the respondent to answer in any way he/she sees fit, while the latter require the respondent to choose from a set of alternatives. Closed-ended questions can be simple 'yes' or 'no' questions, multiple-choice questions, checklist-type questions, 'true' or 'false' questions, and matching questions.

Examples of open-ended questions are as follows:

■ What do you think are some major problems facing health sciences education today?

■ Are there any circumstances in which the use of dagga should be legalised?

Examples of closed-ended questions are as follows:

- Are you male or female?
- Please indicate your annual income level for the previous year with a tick against the appropriate number:
  - ❑ R000,00 to R49 999,99.
  - ❑ R50 000,00 to R99 999,99.
  - ❑ R100 000,00 to R149 999,99.
  - ❑ R150 000,00 or more.

A structured, closed-ended alternative to an open-ended question such as 'What led you to study physiotherapy?' could be 'Your decision to study physiotherapy was mainly determined by

- your parents
- your social environment
- your interest in serving people
- the advantage of earning a salary while studying?'

Open-ended questions are not based on preconceived answers; they are therefore appropriate for explanatory studies, case studies or studies based on qualitative analysis of data. They generally provide richer, more diverse data than can be obtained with the use of closed-ended questions. These questions are also easier to construct, although they take longer to answer, and the very diversity of the answers makes them more difficult for the researcher to code and analyse. Issues of validity and reliability also come to the fore.

Closed-ended questions limit the answers to the options provided by the researcher.

According to Booysen (2003), the greater the complexity of the mental tasks that the respondents are required to perform, the greater amount of visual and other answering aids will help to obtain true answers.

This has several advantages for the researcher. It facilitates the coding and analysing of data. Moreover, respondents are able to complete more closed-ended items in a given amount of time, and they are frequently more willing to complete closed-ended items than they are to compose lengthy responses to open-ended questions. A drawback of closed-ended questions is that they are more difficult to construct than open-ended items. Furthermore, there is the possibility that the researcher may neglect or overlook potentially significant responses. Closed-ended items may also be superficial, and some respondents can become frustrated with the limited responses provided.

In terms of the **words or phrases** that the researcher needs to use when formulating the questions, he/she must pay attention to these guidelines:

- Questions should be *simple* and *short*. Complex questions should be broken up into several simple ones.

- Concomitantly, questions should *not be 'double-barrelled'*, that is, containing two questions. For example: 'Do you plan to pursue a Master' degree in your clinical speciality and seek an administrative position upon graduation?' Such a question should be divided into two separate questions.
- Questions should be *unambiguous*. Words that are too general or too vague, or that could give rise to different interpretations should be replaced with more specific terms. For instance, words such as 'often', 'many' and 'enough' should be replaced by 'three times a week', 'ten', 'two meals a day', and so on. An expression like 'dependent children' should read 'children for whom you are responsible'.
- Questions should be *understandable*. Vocabulary that is adapted to the level of education of the participants should be used. Technical expressions, health care sciences jargon and sophisticated language is inappropriate and should be avoided.
- *Leading questions* should be *avoided*. These are questions that favour one type of answer over another, for example: 'Don't you agree that ...?' and ' ... is it not so?'.
- Questions should be stated in an *affirmative* rather than a negative manner.

The **arrangement** of the questions in a questionnaire is critical. All the questions must be arranged in a way that is logical and relevant to the respondent. There are various strategies that can help you as the researcher:
1 Start with the cover letter. In essence, this is the information leaflet about the study which includes an explanation of how the ethical issues will be dealt with, as well as instructions on how to complete the questionnaire.
2 Group together similar questions or all questions about a certain topic. For example, if you are studying Aids patients' knowledge of the disease, you should group questions about transmission in one section and those concerning treatment in another section.
3 Ask interesting and/or easier questions first.
4 Ask for sensitive information last. It is thought that the respondent is more likely to answer sensitive questions when these are placed at the end of the questionnaire.
5 Arrange the questions from general to specific.
6 Repeat the content of a question, formulated in different ways, in different parts of the questionnaire. This is a method of checking the truthfulness of the answers, in other words, the honesty of the respondent. It is particularly useful for topics about which the respondent may have reason to lie in order to conceal something or to impress you.

In terms of **length**, the questionnaire must be long enough to obtain the necessary information, but not so long that it tires or bores the respondent. It is recommended that questionnaires should take no more than 20 to 25 minutes to complete. A long questionnaire may discourage a response and can prove costly.

When the researcher has drafted the questionnaire, it should be **critically reviewed** by others who are knowledgeable about instrument construction and the content, and by a lay-person who can give meaningful insight based on his/her knowledge of the topic and the sample. The instrument should also be pre-tested with a small sample of respondents, and revised if necessary. A pre-test is a trial run to determine, as far as possible, whether the instrument is clearly worded and free from major biases, and whether it is appropriate for the type of information envisaged.

With regard to its **overall appearance**, a questionnaire should be neat in appearance and grammatically correct, and should *not* contain typing or spelling errors. It should not have a cluttered appearance – the questions should be well spaced and surrounded by adequate margins. An untidy questionnaire that contains errors will not motivate the respondent to address the questions.

There are many methods of **distributing** questionnaires. They can be mailed or delivered by hand, or given in groups, one-on-one or even by computer. Whatever the method, a covering letter should accompany every questionnaire. It may be the single most important factor in motivating respondents to complete the questionnaire. When writing the covering letter, the researcher should try to imagine him-/herself as the recipient. Clear, comprehensive and concise instructions should also be submitted with the questionnaire. And it is helpful to provide respondents with an example of the appropriate way to respond to a particular type of question.

Interviews

The interview is a method of data collection in which an interviewer obtains responses from a subject in a face-to-face encounter, through a telephone call or by electronic means. Interviews are frequently used in exploratory and descriptive research and in case studies. They are the most direct method of obtaining facts from the respondent. They can also be useful in ascertaining values, preferences, interests, tasks, attitudes, beliefs and experience.

Data-collection interviews are generally classified as either 'structured' or 'unstructured'. Most interviews, however, range between the two classifications and are thus referred to as 'semi-structured'.

Structured interviews are formalised so that all respondents hear the same questions in the same order and in the same manner. These interviews are most appropriate when straightforward, factual information is desired. The instrument used here is the interview schedule. The **interview schedule** is a questionnaire with closed-ended or fixed alternative questions, as well as indications of how to answer each question. The interview schedule must be presented to each respondent in exactly the same way. The interviewer is restricted to the provided questions in the order in which they appear on the schedule, with relatively little freedom for deviation. This is done to minimise the role and influence of the interviewer and to enable a more objective comparison of results.

The **unstructured interview** is more free-flowing, with its structure being limited only by the focus of the research. It leaves the wording and organisation of questions, and sometimes even the topic, to the discretion of the interviewer. Unstructured interviews are conducted more like a normal conversation, but with a purpose. They are particularly appropriate for exploratory or qualitative research studies, where the researcher does not possess enough knowledge about the topic to structure questions in advance of data collection. The interviewer may start the interview with a broad opening statement: 'How do you feel about working with people with Aids?' Depending on how the respondent replies, the researcher invites him/her to add information or to clarify the initial response.

Probe follow-ups can be used to increase detailed exploration. **Probes** are prompting questions that encourage the respondent to elaborate on the topic, for example: 'Tell me more about ...', 'What do you mean by ...?', 'Can you describe ...?', 'I am not sure I understand. Could you explain further?' and 'How did you feel then?'. Such probes give the interviewer an opportunity to clarify and expand responses and explicate meaning. They also enhance rapport in that they indicate to the informant that the researcher is truly interested in understanding his/her experience.

Unstructured interviews will produce more in-depth information on the subjects' beliefs and attitudes than can be obtained through any other data-gathering procedure.

The majority of interviews fall somewhere between the structured and unstructured types of interviews. During a **semi-structured interview**, the interviewer must ask a certain number of specific questions, but can also pose additional probes. Both closed-ended and open-ended questions are included in a semi-structured interview.

Focus group interviews are interviews with groups of about 5 to 15 people whose opinions and experiences are requested simultaneously. Apart from the obvious practical advantages, this method is often useful in allowing participants to share their thoughts with each other. In this way, they generate new ideas and consider a range of views before answering the researcher's questions. Focus groups are particularly useful in participatory and action research where members of the community are equal participants in the planning and implementation of the research, and where the topic is a practical community concern. A disadvantage, however, is that some people are uncomfortable talking in groups. The researcher who wants to use focus groups must be skilled at facilitating group discussions.

The development, sequencing and wording considerations of **interview questions** are similar to those related to questionnaires and should be reviewed prior to the interviews. In addition, all interview schedules should be pre-tested and assessed for reliability and validity.

In the case of structured interviews, the data obtained are usually recorded directly onto the interview schedule or on a separate coding sheet. The process of **recording responses** should be absolutely clear to the interviewer. Data obtained from semi-structured and unstructured interviews can be recorded on audiotapes or videotapes. Field notes and logs are frequently the record-keeping devices for interviews.

Training should be provided for all interviewers who will collect data during a study. Training should be carried out in groups, so that every interviewer receives the same instructions. The more unstructured the interview, the more training and experience is required of the interviewers.

All interviews should occur at a time that is convenient for both the researcher and the respondent. Allowing **adequate time** is crucial to the completion of the interview schedules. Moreover, interviews may occur in a variety of **settings**, for example home, ward, clinic or school. Regardless of the setting, the interviewer should attempt to seek as much privacy as possible for the interview.

In face-to-face interviews, the interviewer can have a great deal of **influence on the outcome**. Studies have shown that gender, ethnic origin, manner of speaking and clothing influence the answers provided by respondents. In telephone interviews, the interviewer's verbal mannerisms, such as tone of voice and dialect, can be a positive or negative factor in obtaining cooperation from the respondents.

Scales

These are self-report data-collection instruments that ask respondents to report their attitudes or feelings on a continuum. A scale is composed of a set of numbers, letters or symbols that have rules and that can be used to 'locate' individuals on a continuum. There are different types of scales, the most common being semantic, differential, rating, summated rating, Likert, Guttman and visual analogue.

A **Likert scale** is an example of a summated rating scale which is frequently used to test attitudes or feelings. It is summative in that item scores are added to obtain the final result. It consists of a number of declarative statements about the topic, and five or seven responses for each statement, ranging from 'strongly agree' to 'strongly disagree'. Figure 11.2 provides an example.

Statement 1	Health care professionals should practise therapeutic touch in patient care situations				
	Strongly disagree	Disagree	Uncertain	Agree	Strongly agree
	1	2	3	4	5
Figure 11.2 Example of a Likert scale					

An approximately equal number of positively and negatively worded items should be included in a Likert instrument. To score a Likert scale, the score responses of all items are added to obtain a total score. The values obtained are treated as interval data. If five responses are used, as in Figure 11.2, scores on each item generally range from 1 to 5. If 20 items are included on an instrument, the total score could vary from 20 to 100. A score of 1 is usually given to 'strongly disagree', and a score of 5 to 'strongly agree'. Negatively worded items are often reverse scored, in which case 'strongly disagree' is given a score of 5, and 'strongly agree' a score of 1.

There is far more information in the literature about scales. Should you wish to find out more, consult the references at the end of this book.

Physiological measures

Because of the strong connections between physiological measures and clinical health sciences practice, many researchers use these measures in research. Among the most familiar are blood pressure values, blood values, urine values and electrocardiograms. One of the greatest advantages of physiological measures is their precision and accuracy.

Other techniques

Vignettes

These are short, descriptive sketches of a situation or event to which subjects must respond. For example, Ganong, Coleman and Riley (1988) present hypothetical information about a pregnant woman to two groups of health sciences students in two sessions per group, one a verbal description and the other a videotape of a health care professional interviewing the woman. The information is identical, except that the woman is married in the Group 1 version and unmarried in the Group 2 version. After hearing the verbal report, each group completes two scales. After seeing the videotape, they complete another instrument. The results are interesting. The married woman is rated more favourably than the unmarried woman on all subscales except activity. Furthermore, the students predict that the unmarried woman would have a more difficult time if hospitalised than the married one. Use of the vignettes enables the researcher to distinguish the health care professionals' attitudes about married and unmarried women indirectly. Such an approach is more likely to reveal true attitudes than is a direct question, which often receives an answer that the respondents think is socially desirable.

Records and available data

A researcher need not collect new data to undertake a scientific investigation. These days, researchers are particularly fortunate in the amount and quality of data that is available to them. Hospital records, admission charts, incident reports, care plan statements, students' test and examination results and sick leave records all constitute rich data sources.

Records constitute an economical source of information. They permit an examination of trends over time, and they eliminate the need for the researcher to seek cooperation from participants. However, the use of records may be exposed to many sources of error. The records may contain institutional biases, facts may be distorted, some facts may be omitted, record-keeping may be erratic, the collection of data may have been stopped for political or financial reasons, and some data are not readily available owing to their confidential nature.

Critical incidents

The critical incident technique is used in a variety of ways in health sciences research. It is a set of procedures for collecting direct observations of human behaviour in a way that facilitates potential usefulness in solving practical problems. An incident relates to any observable human activity that is sufficiently complete in itself to permit inferences to be made. For example, health care professionals can be asked to report incidents that they observe which are effective or ineffective in meeting certain goals. A researcher may be interested in establishing factors that relate to giving a good patient report. Health care professionals could be asked to describe activities that result in an effective report being given by the nurse in charge of a ward. Analysis of the responses will enable the researcher to compile a description of effective and ineffective report-giving. In another example, new mothers could be asked to identify the most stressful event that occurred during labour or delivery.

As with all data collection, the collection of critical incidents requires careful preparation, planning and practice.

Summary

In this chapter, we focused on data-collection techniques. We discussed the five important questions that a researcher must pose when planning data collection and explored the most commonly used and some of the less frequently used techniques. We provided the advantages and disadvantages of each technique as, with this knowledge, the researcher should be able to select the most appropriate method for the study at hand.

Exercises

Complete these exercises:

1 You are interested in studying the experiences of young men who are dependent on drugs. Outline what you might do to collect data by means of a highly structured and an unstructured self-report method.

2 An investigation of unemployed health care professionals is to be accomplished by means of a mailed questionnaire. Draft a covering letter to accompany the questionnaire.

3 A researcher is planning to study temper tantrums displayed by hospitalised children. Would you recommend that he/she use a time sampling or an event sampling approach? Justify your choice.

4 What are the steps in instrument development? Describe how error can be reduced in this process.

5 What considerations must the researcher take into account when choosing a self-report method?

6 Find the flaws in the following questions and suggest improvements:
   a) How do you feel about Aids and cancer?
   b) Do you believe that smoking is an unhealthy habit?
   c) Do you often eat sweets?
   d) Do you support the statement made by the head of department at an educational institution that students 'lack a sense of responsibility'?

12 Data quality

LEARNING OUTCOMES

On completion of this chapter, you should be able to demonstrate your understanding of

- the major types of measurement error
- the major sources of measurement error
- instrument validity, and the contrast between four types of validity
- reliability, and a comparison between three types of reliability
- other factors affecting data quality
- a pilot study
- the criteria for evaluating data-collection instruments.

Introduction

In this chapter we pay attention to factors that can affect reliability and validity in data collection. All researchers want to produce quality research. They want the results to be meaningful, to reflect reality as accurately as possible and to be replicable. Unfortunately, all measurement is accompanied by the possibility of error. No data-collection technique is perfect. Therefore, it is important that researchers control for error and reduce error to the lowest possible level.

Types of error

Two types of error can occur in the measurement process: random errors and systematic or constant errors.

Random errors

A random error occurs by chance and is due to random disturbances in performance on the measure. It is an unpredictable error that is unsystematic in nature and that results in inconsistent data. Random errors thus directly affect the reliability of the data. This type of error is caused by factors relating to the subject, the researcher, the environment or the instrument.

Systematic errors

A systematic error, or constant error, consistently affects the measurement of the variable in the same way each time that the measurement is done. This non-random bias impacts on the reliability of a measure. It provides an incorrect measure of the variable, and the error will be the same for every subject. An example of this type of error is a weight scale that consistently weighs a person 1 kg less than is his/her actual body weight. The measurement appears to be reliable, as repeated measures of the same item will result in the same weight. However, the measurement is not a valid one.

Other examples are social desirability, where the research subjects want to please the researcher and constantly answer items in a way that they perceive to be socially desirable, whether or not the answers are actually true; and acquiescent response sets, that is, the subject consistently agrees or disagrees with the questions. These habits are always present in some people, and these people will always bias their responses, to *any* questionnaire or interview. The researcher must take special precaution to design his/her instrument so that such errors can be controlled.

Sources of measurement error

There are many sources of error in research measurement. The most common are those caused by factors of the subject, researcher, environment and instrumentation.

Subject factors

People are a common source of error. A subject who is tired, sick, hungry, angry, irritable or confused, for example, may cause error in the instrumentation. In fact, *any* changing physical, emotional or psychological state of the subject can introduce error into the measurement process. The subject's awareness of a researcher's presence during observation, anonymity of responses in a self-report study and the friendliness of the researcher may also cause bias. The careful researcher ensures that the factors that influence the subject and the subject's responses are controlled.

Researcher factors

The researcher can influence the results of the study in many ways, for example with his/her physical appearance, or his/her clothes, demeanour and personal attributes. In situations where the researcher or data collector is feeling fatigued, impatient, bored, ill or distracted, for example, this state may also contribute to random error. The careful researcher attempts to put aside his/her personal feelings during the data-collection process.

Environmental factors

Many factors that cause random error in measurement can stem from the physical environment in which the research occurs, such as weather, temperature, lighting, noise and interruptions. The careful researcher ensures that the environment is conducive to testing, and that all testing times and sites are similar.

Instrumentation factors

Many factors causing random error have their source in the instrument. For example, unclear questions, unclear directions, inadequate sampling of items, the format of the questions, the order in which questions are asked and the way questions are worded can all be a source of random error. The careful researcher conducts a small-scale or pilot study to find out if other sources become apparent.

Validity of data-collection instruments

In Chapters 8 and 9, we discussed internal and external validity; in this chapter we deal with the related topic of instrument validity. **Instrument validity** seeks to ascertain whether an instrument accurately measures what it is supposed to measure, given the context in which it is applied. Unless the researcher can be sure that the instruments are actually measuring the things they are supposed to be measuring, he/she cannot be certain of what the results mean. For example, if he/she designs a study to examine parenting skills but uses an instrument that actually measures general coping skills, the results of the study are invalid. Similarly, if the researcher examines the relationship between effective health care and a particular kind of education, yet uses an instrument that actually measures attitudes toward health sciences as a profession, the results can be either misleading or meaningless.

We will now discuss the four most common types of validity.

Content validity

Content validity is an assessment of how well the instrument represents all the components of the variable to be measured. When one or more component is neglected, the researcher cannot claim to be measuring whatever he/she is interested in. For example, if the researcher designs a questionnaire on individuals' attitudes to eating but forgets to ask about the significance of food in the subjects' lives, the instrument is incomplete and therefore has poor content validity.

This type of validity is used mainly in the development of questionnaires, inter-view schedules or interview guides. Usually, the researcher who constructs the instrument bases his/her claim on a literature review. Such a review reveals the essential aspects of the variable that must be included in the content. The instrument is then presented to a group of experts in the field for evaluation of the content validity of the instrument. The experts evaluate each item on the instrument with regard to the degree to which the variable to be tested is represented, as well as the instrument's overall suitability for use. In examining the variable, they assess not only that which the instrument measures but also that which it does not measure. Thus the issue is how representative are the questions on the test of the phenomenon under study. The experts do not perform statistical measurements in judging content validity.

Content validity always precedes the actual collection of data.

Face validity

Face validity is the most obvious, and the weakest, kind of instrument validity. It merely means that the instrument appears to measure what it is supposed to measure. It is essentially based on an intuitive judgement made by experts in the field. The researcher may find the procedure useful in the instrument development process with regard to determining readability and clarity of content. However, it should not be considered a satisfactory alternative to other types of validity.

Establishing face and content validity is just the first task in establishing the accuracy of the data-collection instrument. Before using the instrument in a new study, the researcher should seek more objective means of establishing its validity.

Criterion-related validity

This term refers to a pragmatic approach to establish a relationship between the scores on the instrument in question and other external criteria. The researcher can test whether an instrument measures what it is expected to measure by comparing it to another measure that is *known* to be valid. This other measure is called the 'criterion measure'. If the data collected using the instrument in question closely matches the data collected using the criterion measure, then the researcher may conclude that the new instrument is also valid. The two sets of data must be collected from the same group of subjects. A new instrument often needs to be developed even if a valid one already exists because the existing valid tool would neither meet the research aims nor suit its design.

We will now briefly examine the two kinds of criterion-related validity.

Predictive validity

Predictive validity deals with future outcomes. It involves comparing the research instrument results obtained from a particular population to an event or a measure (criterion) that is expected to occur in that population in the future. For example, a health sciences researcher finds evidence in the literature of a relationship between high stress and the onset of illness. He designs an instrument to measure stress in adults 65 years or older, and administers it to a large group of such adults. On the basis of his results, he predicts which persons are more likely to develop illnesses in the coming year. At the end of the year, he is able to determine the accuracy of his prediction by correlating the scores obtained from the stress scale with the onset of illness for the total year in the persons who participated in the study.

Another example is provided by Bless and Higson-Smith (2000). A researcher in an education department has evidence that students' motivation is directly related to their final marks. She develops a questionnaire to measure motivation and administers it to a large group of students. On the basis of her results, she is able to predict which students will do well and which students will do poorly in the final exams. At the end of the year, the students write their final exams and the researcher is able to determine the accuracy of her predictions, based on the students' motivation at the beginning of the year.

A statistical test is done to establish the degree of correlation between the research instrument result and the criterion measure. These tests are discussed in most textbooks on statistics. In cases like these, the difficulty is that the criterion measure may have resulted from variables other than those under investigation. In the above example, study variables such as different textbooks, study habits and circumstances could have influenced the results. Predictive validity should only be used if the researcher is convinced that the variable of concern has a clear criterion measure against which another instrument can be tested.

Concurrent validity

Concurrent validity differs from predictive validity in that the results of the new data-collection instrument are compared to those of a criterion measure at the same point in time. For example, a self-report measure of pain, that is, the new instrument, may be compared with physiological measures of pain, such as pulse rate; or the results of a newly constructed behavioural checklist to measure health care professionals' job satisfaction could be compared with the results of an established job satisfaction instrument shown to be valid for health care professionals. A high correlation between the results of the two dissimilar tests would indicate concurrent validity for the checklist. The main difficulty in practice with criterion-related validity is finding a relevant criterion which is itself valid and reliable. Once the researcher has established a criterion, validity can be measured by correlating the test score and the criterion score.

Construct validity

Construct validity is concerned with this question: 'What construct is the instrument actually measuring?'. It measures the relationship between the instrument and the related theory. This type of validity is the most important and most frequently used of the various forms of validity we have discussed thus far. Construct validity is useful mainly for measures of traits or feelings, such as generosity, anxiety, grief, satisfaction, happiness or pain. It is more complex than criterion-related validity and is usually established over a period of time by several people, instead of by the originator of the instrument alone. It is used to explore the relationship of the instrument's results to measures of the underlying theoretical concept(s) of the instrument.

We will now consider two of the most common approaches used to determine construct validity (Polit & Hungler 1995; Waltz, Strickland & Lenz 1984).

Contrasted groups

Known also as the 'known-groups approach', the contrasted groups approach is carried out by comparing two groups, one of which is known to be extremely 'high' on the concept being measured and the other extremely 'low' on that concept. For example, a group of severely depressed people would be expected to score high on a depression checklist, whereas a group of presumably happy people would score low on that checklist. The checklist, that is, the data-collection instrument, can be given to both groups and the scores can be compared. If the instrument is valid, the mean score of these two groups will be significantly different.

The multi-trait, multi-method approach

This approach is generally regarded as the preferred method of establishing construct validity. This method is based on the two-fold premise that different measures of the same constructs should produce similar results, and that measures of different constructs should produce differing results. To perform this type of validity test, the researcher must have access to more than one method of measuring the construct under study. Anxiety, for example, could be measured by

- observing the subject's behaviour
- asking the subject about his/her anxious feelings
- recording blood-pressure readings
- administering an anxiety inventory.

The results of one of these measures should then be correlated with the results of each of the others in a multi-trait, multi-method matrix (Waltz, Strickland & Lenz 1984).

A variety of data-collection methods, such as self-report observation and collection of physiological data, can be used for testing construct validity. A second requirement of the multi-trait, multi-method approach is that the researcher also measures constructs from which he/she wishes to differentiate the key construct using the same measuring methods. For example, he/she wants to distinguish anxious persons from calm persons. The two concepts are related; the researcher would therefore expect, on average, that persons who exhibited a high degree of anxiety would score extremely low in terms of calmness. The point of including both concepts in a single validation study is to gather evidence that the two concepts are in fact distinct, rather than being two different labels for the same trait or characteristic.

Several other approaches for determining construct validity are described in the literature.

Validity of qualitative data

By their very nature, qualitative research methods do not lend themselves well to statistical calculations of validity. However, this does not imply that qualitative researchers are not concerned with the quality of their data-collection techniques. The central question that determines the concept of validity and reliability addresses the issue of whether the measures used by the researcher yield data that reflect the truth. A number of authors focusing on qualitative research methods suggest strategies that the researcher can employ in data collection to enhance the truthfulness or validity of qualitative results. We deal with several such strategies in Chapter 9.

Reliability of data-collection instruments

Reliability of the research instrument is a further major concern of the researcher when collecting data. 'Reliability' refers to the degree to which the instrument can be depended upon to yield consistent results if used repeatedly over time on the same person, or if used by two researchers. The reliability of an instrument is indicated by a correlation measure which varies between 0 and 1. The nearer the measure is to 1, the higher the correlation.

We will now discuss the three characteristics of reliability that are commonly evaluated.

Stability

Stability of a research instrument refers to its consistency over time. Stability is measured by giving the same individuals an instrument on two occasions within a relatively short period of time and examining their responses for similarities. This method is termed 'test-retest'. Problems with the test-retest technique include the fact that some persons may respond to the instrument the second time on the basis of their memory of their first exposure to it. They may also undergo changes, particularly if the period of intervention is long.

The technique is used in interviewing and in questionnaires. When observations are used, the test of stability is called 'repeated observation'.

Internal consistency

Sometimes also referred to as 'homogeneity', internal consistency addresses the extent to which all items on an instrument measure the same variable. This type of reliability is appropriate only when the instrument is examining one concept or construct at a time. For example, if the instrument is designed to measure assertiveness, all of the items on the instrument must consistently measure assertiveness. Other concepts frequently measured in health sciences are job satisfaction, depression, self-esteem and autonomy.

The common method employed to estimate internal consistency is the split-half method. This is done by splitting the items on the instrument into two halves, and computing correlations between their scores. The halves can be divided by obtaining the scores on the first half of the test and comparing them with the scores on the second half of the test, or by comparing odd-numbered items to even-numbered items. Because the reliability of a measure is associated with the number of items, the split-half procedure tends to decrease the correlation coefficient.

Special statistical tests have been developed to provide measures of internal consistency for questionnaires. Crohnbach's alpha coefficient is the test most frequently used to establish internal consistency. While it is useful for establishing reliability in a highly structured quantitative data-collection instrument, it is far less effective in open-ended questionnaires or interviews, unstructured observations, projective tests, available data, or other qualitative data-collection methods and instruments.

Equivalence reliability

Tests of equivalence attempt to determine whether similar tests given at the same time yield the same results, or whether the same results can be obtained by using different observers at the same time. The former case is frequently referred to as the use of 'parallel forms'. The use of parallel forms requires the availability of alternative versions of a test or questionnaire examining the same concept. The researcher then administers the two instruments consecutively to the same subjects, and compares the results of the two tests statistically to determine the degree of association or correlation between them. This method is more commonly used in educational testing than in health sciences research. However, it may be a useful approach in establishing the reliability of results obtained from knowledge-testing procedures when client-teaching methods are being investigated.

The latter case is frequently referred to as 'inter-rater reliability'. This is the method of testing for equivalence when the design calls for observations. A reliable instrument should produce the same results if both observers are using it in the same way.

Relationship between reliability and validity

Reliability and validity are closely related. The researcher needs to consider both of these qualities when selecting a research instrument. There is no point in using an instrument that is not valid, however reliable it may be. By the same token, if an instrument measures a phenomenon of importance but the measurements are not consistent, it is of no use. In essence, reliability is a part of validity in that an instrument that does not yield reliable results cannot be considered valid. It is possible that an instrument can be used to collect reliable data, but reliability of the method does not guarantee that the data collected are valid measures of the research concepts.

The important skill in developing or finding good measurement techniques involves being able to recognise a technique that is adequate in terms of *both* validity and reliability.

Other factors affecting data quality

In addition to reliability and validity, the researcher must examine a number of other criteria before using a data-collection instrument.

Sensitivity

The 'sensitivity' of an instrument refers to the ability of that instrument to discriminate. In addition, a sensitive instrument can detect change. Therefore, when evaluating data-collection instruments, the evaluator should question if the instrument is sufficiently sensitive to ensure that valid data are collected.

Efficiency

An efficient instrument is one that requires minimum effort and expense, and yet manages to measure with validity and reliability. A questionnaire or interview schedule should only be as long and as complex as is necessary to achieve credible reliability and validity. A perfect instrument that is too complex and too expensive to use will not collect much data. Both the researcher's and research subjects' time should be considered valuable. The cost of various techniques should be weighed. Only information that is necessary for the research should be solicited.

Appropriateness

'Appropriateness' refers to the extent to which the research subjects can meet the demands imposed by the instrument. The content of the instrument should be understood by the researcher and all research subjects. Furthermore, the instrument should be appropriate for the research subjects in terms of their ability and readiness to furnish the required data. Age, literacy level, health status, culture and language are all pertinent considerations. English spoken as a second language, for example, may not always be appropriate in the study of members of ethnic groups who have different first languages.

Ability to generalise

This refers to the expectations of the researcher that instruments that are reliable and valid in one study will be found to be so in another. Previously used instruments found to be reliable are often found to be less so when used on other kinds of groups. For example, an instrument tested for validity and reliability with undergraduate students would not necessarily be valid for use with hospitalised adolescents.

The pilot study

In order to test the practical aspects of a research study, the researcher can conduct a pilot study. Sometimes also referred to as a 'preliminary study', this is a small-scale study conducted prior to the main study on a limited number of subjects from the population at hand. Its purpose is to investigate the feasibility of the proposed study and to detect possible flaws in the data-collection instruments, such as ambiguous instructions or wording, inadequate time limits, and so on, as well as whether the variables defined by operational definitions are actually observable and measurable. Such a pilot study is especially useful if the researcher has compiled the measuring instrument specifically for the purposes of the research project. The time and effort expended in conducting a pilot study are well spent, as pitfalls and errors that may prove costly in the actual study can be identified and avoided.

Measurement evaluation

It is essential that the measurement methods described in a research study are evaluated. The thoroughness and appropriateness of the measurement assessment are critical to the results of the study. If the measures used in the study are flawed, or if insufficient precautions have been taken to avoid errors, the findings are not likely to be meaningful.

A checklist for evaluating the measurement aspects of quantitative and qualitative studies is as follows:

1   Are the conceptual and operational definitions of the variables appropriate and strongly related?

Quantitative data

2   Are the instruments for data collection clearly described and are there any indications in the report of efforts the researcher made to minimise errors?

3   How did the researcher assess the reliability of the data-collection methods? Is/are the method(s) used clearly described and appropriate for the study or should an alternative method have been used? Is the reliability adequate?

4   How was validity assessed? Was/were the method(s) used appropriate for the study or should an alternative method have been used? Does the validity of the instrument appear to be adequate?

5   Were the statistical procedures used to assess the reliability and validity of the study reported in enough detail for the reader?

Qualitative data

6   Are the efforts that the researcher made to enhance or evaluate the trustworthiness of the data discussed clearly and in sufficient detail? If not, is there any other information that allows researchers to conclude that the data are believable?

7   Which precautions did the researcher use and what strategies did he/she employ to enhance or evaluate the trustworthiness of the data? How adequate were the procedures? Could alternative procedures have been used more profitably?

8   How much faith can be placed in the results of the study, based on the information given by the researcher?

Summary

In this chapter, we presented an overview of the factors that may affect the quality of data collected in a research study. Few, if any, measuring instruments are infallible – we explained how errors can occur in studies. We discussed several methods for assessing reliability and validity, and briefly described other factors affecting data quality. Having provided an overview of the pilot study as the method for testing the practical aspects of a study, including its feasibility, the chapter ended with a checklist that the researcher can use to evaluate the measurement aspects of a study.

Exercises

Complete these exercises:

1 The following research descriptions refer to research which may yield unreliable data:

'The satisfaction with regard to service of hospital patients on the day of their discharge.'

'The attitudes of subjects towards different ethnic groups, when some of the questions come from the ethnic groups themselves.'

'The use of an instrument developed for first year students on hospitalised teenagers.'

a) From these descriptions indicate which factors may be responsible for the unreliability.

b) How could reliability be enhanced in each of the examples?

2 Identify some examples of concurrent validity and predictive validity related to research in health sciences practice.

3 Explain what the multi-trait, multi-method of construct validity measures.

13 Data analysis

LEARNING OUTCOMES

On completion of this chapter, you should be able to demonstrate your understanding of

■ data analysis strategies for quantitative and qualitative research studies

■ the broad classifications of statistics

■ the appropriate descriptive statistics to use in presenting selected data

■ the purposes of inferential statistics

■ selected statistical tests used in analysing data from health sciences research.

Introduction

In this chapter, we focus on what to do with the data once they have been collected. It would be impractical for the researcher to try to list individually each piece of collected data. Therefore, he/she must choose methods of organising the raw data and displaying them in a fashion that will provide answers to the research questions. This phase or step is usually referred to as 'data analysis'. **Data analysis** entails categorising, ordering, manipulating and summarising the data and describing them in meaningful terms.

There are various analysis strategies. At present, research studies generally use either narrative or statistical strategies, in conjunction with graphic or pictorial strategies. The type of strategy depends on the research design, the types of variables, the method of sampling and the method by which the data were collected and measured. A descriptive or qualitative research design, or unstructured questions in other designs, often elicit qualitative data of considerable depth. The narrative strategy would be the strategy of choice for analysing such data. Data collected by means of quantitative designs may use strategies also used in qualitative analysis and, in addition, may use statistical strategies.

Table 13.1 summarises the suitable analysis strategies for different types of data and levels of enquiry.

Table 13.1 Analysis strategies arranged by level of enquiry and type of data

| Type of data | Purpose of analysis | | | |
	Description Levels 1–2	Association/ Differences Levels 2–3	Patterns of relationships Levels 2–4	Hypothesis testing Levels 3–8
Qualitative (words or images)	Narrative Graphic	Narrative Graphic	Narrative Graphic	Not applicable
Quantitative (numbers) Nominal	Narrative Graphic Statistical	Narrative Graphic Statistical	Narrative Graphic	Graphic Statistical
Ordinal	Narrative Graphic Statistical	Narrative Graphic Statistical	Graphic Statistical	Graphic Statistical
Interval	Graphic Statistical	Graphic Statistical	Graphic Statistical	Statistical

Source: Adapted from Roberts and Burke (1989: 277)

These strategies are not mutually exclusive; in other words, by using one method the researcher does not prevent him-/herself from using another. He/she can use them together to make a stronger case in answering the research question. Furthermore, you should not see the suggestions in Table 13.1 as absolute. A researcher's preference, which is based on his/her philosophical leaning, training and experience, will often influence the choice of strategy. However, it is important for the researcher to bear in mind that if the analysis strategy is not logically consistent with the level of enquiry and with the level of the data, the answers to the questions will be flawed and the usefulness of the results will be doubtful. The researcher must also remember that data analysis must be planned before the data are collected. Without a plan, the researcher may collect data that is unsuitable, insufficient or excessive; and he/she may not know what to do with them.

Analysis of quantitive data

The most powerful tool available to the researcher in analysing quantitative data is *statistics*. With regard to Table 13.1, notice that statistical strategies are recommended for all quantitative data, with the exception of nominal data, in which the purpose of the research is to establish patterns of relationships. Moreover, quantitative data is classified according to the level of measurement or measurement scale into nominal, ordinal and interval. The ratio level is omitted because both interval and ratio data use the same types of statistical analysis, and we deal with these levels of measurement in Chapter 11.

Without the aid of statistics, the quantitative data would be simply a chaotic mass of numbers. Statistical methods enable the researcher to reduce, summarise, organise, manipulate, evaluate, interpret and communicate quantitative data.

Descriptive statistics are used to describe and summarise data. They convert and condense a collection of data into an organised, visual representation, or picture, in a variety of ways, so that the data have some meaning for the readers of the research report. A descriptive approach employs measures such as frequency distributions, measures of central tendency and dispersion or variability, and measures of relationships.

Inferential statistics use sample data to make an inference about the population of the study at hand. They permit the researcher to infer that particular characteristics in a sample exist in the larger population. They also help the researcher to determine whether the difference that is found between two groups, such as an experimental and a control group, is a genuine difference, or whether it is merely a 'chance difference' that occurs because a non-representative sample is chosen from the population. In an inferential approach, P values – that is, the probability that the outcome is owing to chance – are used to communicate the significance or lack thereof of the data. Furthermore, inferential statistics facilitate the testing of hypotheses. Such statistics include the chi-square test, t-test, analysis of variance, analysis of co-variance, factor analysis and multi-variate analysis.

We will now explore these two categories of statistical methods in greater detail.

Descriptive statistics

Descriptive statistics describe and synthesise data. These statistics can be subdivided into groups according to the summary functions that they perform. We now provide an overview of five groups of these statistics, referring to simple formulae and calculations. You can find more detail on these measures in any handbook on statistics.

Frequency distributions

'Frequency' refers to the number of times that a result occurs. Frequencies are obtained by simply counting the occurrence of scores or values represented in the data. A **frequency distribution** is a systematic arrangement of the lowest to the highest scores linked with the number of times the score occurs. Each score can be listed separately, or the results can be grouped. This means that the results are subdivided into classes, or collections of scores, which are grouped together. The extent of a class is determined by its boundaries.

For example, when classifying according to age, the classes may be 0–9, 10–19, 20–29, etc. The class 0–9 reflects the number of children up to nine years of age, the class of 10–19 reflects the numbers of individuals whose ages range from 10 to 19, and so on. It is vitally important that classes are mutually exclusive and do not overlap. In the age classification, for example, the classes should not be 0–10, 10–20, 20–30, etc.

Frequency distributions are appropriate for interval and ratio data. Frequency counts are appropriate for nominal and ordinal data, and are obtained by counting the occurrence of each observation in a category.

Examples of organising data according to level of measurement

We will now examine some examples of the organisation of data according to level of measurement.

Example 1: Nominal data

In the case of *nominal data*, a researcher is interested in investigating whether more men than women suffering from Aids were admitted to hospital X in 2004. The investigation involves counting the number of cases falling into each gender category. If there were 50 patients, of whom 10 were male and 40 female, the data could be presented as shown in Table 13.2 on the next page, which displays the following conventions in tabulating data:

- The table as a whole and the categories must be clearly and fully labelled so that the readers can unambiguously interpret what they are observing.
- The label *f* represents frequency of cases or measurements falling into a given category.
- The label **n** represents the total number of cases or measurements in a sample.
- The label **N** represents the number of cases in a population.

Table 13.2 Frequency count of gender of patients with Aids admitted to hospital X during 2004	
Gender	Frequency (f)
Males (M)	10
Females (F)	40
	n = **50**

Example 2: Ordinal data
In the case of *ordinal data*, the data are represented by counting the number of cases, or the frequency, of each ordered rank making up a scale. A co-researcher is involved in a project to evaluate the efficacy of a new analgesic versus traditional treatment. A post-test-only control group design is used. The experimental group receives the analgesic and the control group the traditional treatment. Twenty patients are randomly assigned to each group. Pain intensity is assessed by the patient's pain reports five hours after minor surgery, on the following scale:

5 – excruciating pain
4 – severe pain
3 – moderate pain
2 – mild pain
1 – no pain

The raw data are as follows:
- Experimental group: 3, 4, 5, 3, 3, 3, 4, 2, 1, 3, 2, 1, 3, 4, 5, 2, 3, 3, 3, 3.
- Control group: 5, 4, 4, 4, 5, 3, 4, 3, 2, 4, 4, 2, 4, 5, 3, 4, 4, 4, 5, 5.

Once the results have been tallied, the above data can be presented in a frequency table as shown in Table 13.3 on the next page. This demonstrates that once the data have been tabulated, the outcome of the investigation can be seen. In this example, the pain reported by the experimental group is less than that of the control group. When tallying raw data, it is helpful to use the familiar 'gate method' of recording

Pain intensity	Experimental groups (Analgesic) F	Control group (Traditional) F
1	2	–
2	3	2
3	10	3
4	3	10
5	2	5
	n = 20	n = 20

Table 13.3 Reported pain intensity of patients following traditional and new analgesic treatments

frequencies. Four vertical lines are listed for the first four occurrences of a score, and a slash is used to indicate the fifth occurrence. This procedure is repeated until all scores are recorded.

Example 3: Interval or ratio data

In the case of *interval or ratio data*, we use the example of patients who are routinely weighed on admission to hospital. The researcher must summarise the weights of 50 female patients who were admitted to a female medical ward over a specific period of time. The weights, which are the raw data, are as follows (to nearest kilogram):

75, 67, 76, 71, 73, 86, 72, 77, 80, 75, 80, 96, 93
75, 73, 83, 81, 82, 73, 92, 81, 87, 76, 84
78, 79, 99, 100, 88, 77, 71, 76, 75, 83, 66, 79
95, 85, 77, 87, 90, 73, 72, 68, 84, 69, 78, 77, 84, 94

Once the results have been tallied, they can be presented in a frequency table as shown in Table 13.4.

It is easier to understand the data by studying Table 13.4 than by looking at the raw data.

Evidently, frequency distributions and frequency counts present useful summaries of data, as they provide the reader with a much clearer picture of the results than that provided by the raw scores.

Table 13.4 Grouped frequency distribution of patients' weight in a given ward

Class interval	f
96–100	3
91–95	4
86–90	5
81–85	9
76–80	13
71–75	12
66–70	4
	n = 50

Simple descriptive statistics

Once the data have been summarised in a frequency distribution, it is often useful to make comparisons concerning the relative frequencies of scores falling into specific categories. Simple descriptive statistics used for this purpose are ratios, proportions, percentages and rates.

Ratios are statistics which express the relative frequency of one set of frequencies, 'A', in relation to another, 'B'. The formula for ratio is as follows:

$$\text{Ratio} = \frac{A}{B}$$

Therefore, the ratio of males to females for the data presented in Table 13.2 is as follows:

$$\text{Ratio (males to females)} = \frac{10}{40} \quad 0{,}25$$

$$\text{Ratio (females to males)} = \frac{40}{10} \quad 4{,}0$$

Ratios are useful in the health sciences when we are interested in the distribution of illnesses or symptoms, or in the categories of subjects requiring or benefiting from treatment. The ratio calculated above tells us about the relative frequency of Aids admissions for males and females.

A **proportion** is a part of a whole, and is calculated by putting the frequency of one category over that of the total numbers in the sample or population. For example, if a cake is cut into eight equal slices, each slice is a proportion and can be written as $\frac{1}{8}$ or 0,125. In the example presented in Table 13.2 the proportion of males is as follows:

$$\frac{10}{50\,(10+40)} = \frac{1}{5} \text{ or } 0{,}2$$

A **percentage** is the number of parts per 100 that a certain portion of the whole represents. Proportions can be transformed into percentages by multiplying by 100. In the previous example, the percentage of males admitted with Aids would be:

$0,2 \times 100 = 20\%$

In the example on pain intensity, the percentage of people experiencing excruciating pain in the experimental groups in Table 13.3 is as follows:

$$\frac{2}{20} \times 100 = 10\%$$

The two **rates** commonly used in epidemiological studies are *incidence rates* and *prevalence rates*. When summarising the results of an epidemiological investigation, it is common for the researcher to compare the number of cases of the disease with the size of the population at risk of having the disease. He/she does this by calculating rates.

The *incidence rate* of a disease over a period of time is as follows:

$$\frac{\text{number of new cases over the period}}{\text{population at risk}}$$

For example, in town X the number of new cases of diabetes in 2004 was 289. The total number of people suffering from diabetes on 30 June 2004 was 3 492. The population of town X at the time was 176 000.

Thus, the incidence rate for diabetes per 100 000 is:

$$\frac{289}{176\ 000} \times 100\ 000 = 164,2$$

The *prevalence rate* of a disease at a point in time is as follows:

$$\frac{\text{total number of cases of the disease at that time}}{\text{population at risk}}$$

The prevalence rate of diabetes per 100 000 people from town X on 30 June 2004 is:

$$\frac{3\ 492}{176\ 000} \times 100\ 000 = 1984,1$$

All five of these simple descriptive statistics were obtained by the mathematical manipulation of raw data. Thus, all of these statistics are useful for summarising such data.

Measures of central tendency

In many cases the condensing or summarising of data is not of as much interest or importance as the average value of a distribution. Measures of central tendency are statistics or numbers expressing the most typical or average scores in a distribution. The mean, median and mode are measures of central tendency.

The **mean** is the arithmetical average of all the scores in a distribution. To obtain the mean, the researcher adds all the scores together and divides the total by the total number of scores. For example, the researcher assesses levels of pain and obtains the following six scores on the pain scale: 12, 17, 14, 5, 12, 3. The mean would be as follows:

$$\frac{63 \quad \text{(the sum of all the scores)}}{6 \quad \text{(the total number of scores)}} \quad \text{or} \quad 10{,}5$$

The mean is appropriate for interval and ratio data. It is considered the most stable measure of central tendency for these levels of data if the distribution is normal. If the distribution is not normal, the mean will not present an accurate picture of the distribution.

The **median** is the midpoint score or value in a group of data ranked from lowest to highest. Half of the scores are above the median and half of the scores are below. If the number of scores or values is uneven, that is, odd, the median is the middle score or value. If the number of scores or values is even, the median is the midpoint between the two middle values and is found by averaging these two values. If the pain scores, which are used for calculating the mean, are ranked, the result is as follows:

3   5   12   12   14   17

The median for these scores is as follows:

$$\frac{12 + 12}{2} = 12$$

The median is the best value of central tendency for ordinal data. It is also appropriate for interval and ratio data. It presents a more accurate picture of such data when the distribution is curved than would be presented by the mean.

The **mode** is the value or score that occurs most frequently in a distribution. For example, in the example of scores on the pain scale, 12 is the score that occurs most frequently. Hence, the mode is 12. If a distribution has only one mode, as in the example, it is referred to as 'unimodal'. If there are two modes, the distribution is referred to as 'bimodal'. If there are more than two modes, it is referred to as 'multimodal'. The mode can be used with every level of measurement. Although it is not the best measure of central tendency, it is the most appropriate measure for nominal data.

Measures of variability

Measures of variability describe how widespread values or scores are in a distribution. While the mean, median and mode describe something about the middle of a set of numbers, the variation among the numbers shows whether or not the scores cluster around the middle with few scores at either extreme. The three statistics commonly used to indicate the numerical value of variability are the range, the variance and the standard deviation.

The **range** is the simplest method for examining variation among scores and refers to the difference between the smallest and largest value in a distribution. Using the pain scores example, the total range would be 17 minus 3, or 14. Clearly, the range is affected by extreme cases and gives no indication of what lies between the highest and lowest scores. The range can be used with ordinal, interval and ratio data. However, its usefulness is limited, because one extreme score can change the range drastically.

The **variance** is defined as the sum of the squared deviations about the mean divided by the total number of values. It is an intermediate value that is used in calculating the standard deviation.

The **standard deviation** is the most widely used measure of variability when interval or ratio data are described. It indicates how values vary about the mean of the distribution, and is defined as the square root of the variance. Two sets of results with the same mean may differ considerably in distribution, but the standard deviation quantifies this difference. The larger the standard deviation, the more spread out the scores are about the mean in a distribution. Textbooks on statistics provide a variety of calculable formulae to derive these statistics. Furthermore, the widespread use of computers and calculators makes a discussion of these formulae superfluous.

The **normal curve** or **normal distribution** is a special kind of curve that represents the theoretical distribution of population scores. With regard to the curve, 'normal' is a mathematical term used in the sense that a normal distribution of variables is frequently found in biological, behavioural and clinical sciences. Variables such as blood pressure, height and weight are normally distributed in the population. For example, while a few very short and a few very tall people do exist, most people are within a few centimetres of each other in height.

For a frequency curve to approximate the normal curve, a fairly large number of values is needed, that is, at least 30. The normal curve is bell-shaped and symmetrical with maximum height at the mean. The mean, median and mode are equal. Most of the values cluster around the mean. A few values occur on both extremes of the distribution curve. An additional characteristic of the normal curve is that a fixed percentage of the scores falls within a given distance of the mean.

As depicted in Figure 13.1 on the next page, the following always holds true for a normal distribution:

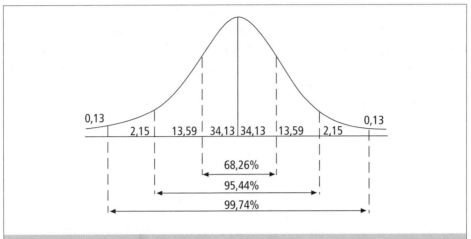

Figure 13.1 Percentage of the normal distribution between the mean and major points

- Approximately 68,26% of observations are located between the mean and one standard deviation on either side of it.
- Approximately 95,44% are located within two standard deviations of the mean on either side of it.
- Approximately 99,74% of observations are within approximately three standard deviations of the mean.
- This leaves 0,26% beyond three standard deviations, that is, 0,13 on either side.

What makes the normal distribution curve so useful is that in research on any normally distributed phenomenon the researcher can use the properties of the curve for making inferences and testing hypotheses. Once the mean and standard deviation of the data set are known, it is possible for him/her to determine precisely the proportion of observations lying between any two values.

In order to make comparisons between groups, standard scores rather than raw scores can be used. Once the mean and standard deviation for a given distribution have been calculated, any raw score can be transformed into a standard, or Z score. The standard score represents by how many standard deviations a specific score is above or below the mean. A Z score of 1,5 means that it is 1,5 standard deviations *above* the mean, whereas a score of –2 means that the observation is 2 standard deviations *below* the mean. By utilising Z scores, the researcher can compare results from scales that utilise different units, such as height and weight.

Measures of relationship

Measures of relationship concern the correlation between variables. The concept of correlation is used when the researcher wants to determine the nature and extent of the relationship between variables. For example, he/she wishes to establish the relationship between weight gain over a six-month period and the average daily calorie intake among a group of diabetics, or between the amount of time spent with a patient and the number of requests for pain medication made by the patient during that time. These data would be gathered on a group of patients. The researcher would want to know whether the two variables vary together. He/she needs to ask him-/herself: 'When diabetics increase their calorie intake, do they or do they not gain weight?' or 'When the time spent with the patient increases, does the amount of the patient's requests for pain medication increase or decrease?'.

There are several ways to examine relationships such as these. We will now briefly explore correlation coefficients, scattergrams and contingency tables.

A **correlation coefficient** is a descriptive statistic or number that expresses the magnitude and direction of the association between two variables. In order to demonstrate that two variables are correlated, the researcher must obtain measures on both variables for the same subjects or events. In the above example, he/she obtains measures of the diabetic patients' weight over a period of time, for example six months, and their calorie intake over the same period.

Several types of correlation coefficients are used in statistics. Those commonly used are as follows:

Φ phi	– when both variables are measured on a nominal scale
ρ (rho) or Spearman's rank	– when both variables are measured on or transformed to ordinal scales
r or Pearson's correlation coefficient	– when both variables are measured on an interval or ratio scale

All of the correlation coefficients listed above are appropriate for quantifying linear relationships between variables. There are other correlation coefficients, such as *eta*, which are used for quantifying non-linear relationships. However, a discussion of the use and calculation of all correlation coefficients is beyond the scope of this book. You can consult statistical texts for further information.

Regardless of which correlation coefficient the researcher employs, these statistics share the following characteristics:
- Correlation coefficients are calculated from pairs of measurements on variables X and Y for the same group of individuals.
- A positive correlation is denoted by +, that is, a plus sign, and a negative correlation by –, that is, a minus sign. A positive correlation means that the two variables tend to increase or decrease together. A negative correlation denotes an

inverse relationship and indicates that as one variable increases the other variable decreases.

- The values of the correlation coefficient range from +1 to −1, where +1 implies a perfect positive correlation, 0 implies no correlation and −1 implies a perfect negative correlation.

To obtain a visual representation of the relationship between the two variables, the researcher plots the values obtained on a scattergram. A **scattergram** is a graphic presentation of the paired scores for each subject on the two variables. Pairs of scores are plotted on a graph by placing dots to indicate where each pair of Xs and Ys intersect. If the pattern of dots extends from the lower left corner to the upper right corner, a positive correlation is indicated. If the dots are distributed from the upper left corner down towards the lower right corner, a negative correlation is said to exist. When the dots are scattered all over the graph, there is an indication that no relation exists between the two variables. The scattergrams in Figure 13.2 illustrate the different correlations.

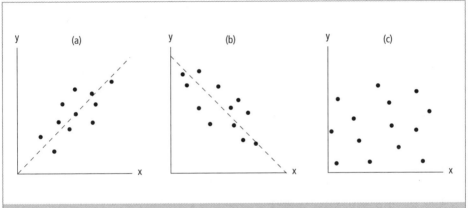

Figure 13.2 Scattergrams representing a) a positive, b) a negative, and c) a case of no relationship between two variables

If data are nominal, relationships cannot be depicted on a scattergram. No actual scores are available in nominal data; rather, frequencies of the occurrence of the values are presented. A **contingency table**, also called a 'cross-tabulation table', is a means of visually displaying the relationship between sets of nominal data. For example, the researcher wishes to determine whether or not there is a relationship between gender and smoking. Table 13.5 on the next page depicts the data that were gathered on 50 male and 50 female subjects. Table 13.5 is called a 2 × 2 contingency table because there are two variables, and each variable has two categories. If smoking had been divided into three categories – such as a) 'never smoke', b) 'smoke

Table 13.5 A 2 × 2 contingency table

Gender	Smoke regularly	Do not smoke regularly	Total
Males	30	20	50
Females	25	25	50
Total	55	45	100

occasionally' and c) 'smoke frequently' – the table would have been called a 2 × 3 table.

The data in Table 13.5 seem to indicate that more men smoke than women. Further calculations must be done to determine whether or not the relationship between these variables is significant. The chi-square statistic is the statistic which would be calculated in this case.

As we have mentioned, if researchers want to describe and summarise the data they have obtained, they will use descriptive statistics. If they want to infer or draw conclusions about something, they will use inferential statistics.

Inferential statistics

We will now consider the two kinds of inferential statistical tests, parametric and non-parametric.

Parametric statistics

Parametric statistics are applied to data where the following underlying assumptions have been made:

- The variables of concern must be normally distributed within the targeted population.
- The selected sample must be representative of the target population.
- The variables are measured by an interval or ratio scale.
- The variances of groups compared should be approximately the same.
- The tests require estimates of parameters, for example mean and standard deviation.

The most common parametric statistical tests used in health sciences research are the t-test and analysis of variance.

The **t-test** is used when the researcher wishes to compare the means of two groups in order to determine whether the differences between the means are significant or caused by chance. There are two forms of t-test – one is used with independent samples, and the other with dependent samples. Samples are independent when there are two separate groups, such as an experimental and a control group, and there is no association between their scores. Samples are dependent when the participants from the two groups are paired in some manner. For example, when the same participants are assessed on a given characteristic before and after an intervention, the sample is considered dependent. Dependent data are also obtained if each subject in one group is matched with a subject in another group on some variable, such as age or weight. The form of the t-test that is used with a dependent sample may be termed 'paired dependent', 'matched' or 'correlated'. Separate formulae are used to calculate the independent t-test and the dependent t-test. You can find these in statistical textbooks.

Analysis of variance (ANOVA) is an extension of the t-test, which permits the researcher to compare more than two means simultaneously. ANOVA uses variances to calculate a value that reflects the differences between two or more means. When using ANOVA, the researcher calculates an F statistic or ratio. The larger the F value, the greater the variation or difference *between* the groups compared with the variation *within* the groups. If a statistically significant difference is found, other tests – called 'post-hoc comparisons', for example Sheffe's or Tukey's tests – can be used to determine which of the means differ significantly.

There is a variety of other parametric statistical tests available for analysing the significance of the obtained data. If you are interested in learning more, you can consult the more advanced research textbooks and statistical texts.

Non-parametric statistics

Non-parametric statistics are sometimes also referred to as 'distribution-free' statistical tests since they are applied to data where no assumptions are made regarding the normal distribution of the targeted population. These statistics are usually applied when the variables have been measured on a nominal or ordinal scale. The chi-square is one of the most widely used non-parametric statistical tests in health sciences research. It is appropriate for comparing sets of data that are in the form of frequencies. Other examples of non-parametric tests are the Mann-Whitney test, which is an alternative to the independent form of the t-test; the Wilcoxon test for correlated samples, which is an alternative to the dependent form of the t-test; and the Kruskal-Wallis test, which is an alternative to ANOVA for comparing significant differences between several groups.

When using inferential statistical techniques to test a hypothesis, the researcher must be well acquainted with several statistical concepts, such as the probability or p value or level of significance, degrees of freedom, critical values, one-tailed and two-tailed tests of significance, and type I and type II errors. You can consult statistical textbooks for clarification of these terms.

In order to choose the most appropriate inferential procedure for a study, the researcher must consider several factors. Some of the more important are as follows:

- Am I testing for differences or for relationships?
- What is the level of measurement of the variables – nominal, ordinal, interval or ratio?
- Does the level of measurement permit the use of parametric statistics?
- What is the size of the sample?
- How many groups or sets of scores are being compared?
- Are the observations or scores dependent or independent?

Use of graphics

As Figure 13.1 illustrates, in addition to statistical tests, the use of graphic displays is recommended for almost every type of data. Graphics can effectively convey information related to data collected in a study, and can be constructed in various ways. They have visual appeal that may cause the reader to analyse the data more closely than would be the case if a written description of the data were presented. To be of value, graphics must be accurate, simple, clear and readily understood by the reader. They should accurately represent the ideas and data presented in the research report. Graphs should also fit the type of data collected; for example, bar charts and pie diagrams are generally used for nominal data, and a histogram and frequency polygon for interval and ratio data. Information on the various types of graphs and how to plot them can be obtained in any statistical textbook.

Analysis of qualitative data

The data in qualitative research is non-numerical, usually in the form of written words or videotapes, audiotapes and photographs. Analysis of data in qualitative studies therefore involves an examination of words rather than the numbers that are considered in quantitative studies. Frequently, a massive amount of data in the form of words is gathered, which makes analysis extremely time consuming. Researchers using qualitative approaches tend to spend hours reflecting on the possible meanings and relationships of the data. This type of analysis is described as a 'hands-on process' during which the researcher becomes deeply immersed in the data; it is also sometimes referred to as 'dwelling' with the data.

Generally, data analysis is not a distinct step in the qualitative research studies process, but is done concurrently with data collection – unlike quantitative research analysis, which does not begin until all the data have been collected. The different forms of qualitative approaches have different forms of analysis. Nevertheless, many qualitative researchers use a series of common steps for analysing their data which begins at the start of the data-collection phase. Typical steps are coding for themes and categories, making memos about the context of and variations in the phenomenon under study, verifying the selected themes through reflection on the data and discussion with other researchers or experts in the field, refining the categories, recording of support data for categories and identifying propositions.

Coding and categorising are generally initiated as soon as data collection begins. Coding is used to organise data collected in interviews and other types of documents. The researcher can check the reliability of the coding by having another person encode the same data and then by checking for agreement. Some researchers validate findings with their subjects and/or other forms of evidence. Developing categories is facilitated through the use of either manual or computer activity.

Manual analysis involves a thorough review of all recorded information that the researcher has obtained during the course of the data collection. If the margin is sufficiently wide, the coding of data can take place on the page itself. Coding involves inventing and applying a category system. For example, with regard to a participant who has been hospitalised for six weeks and who gives an account of her perceptions of hospitalisation, the researcher could classify her statements into types of people described, feelings expressed, levels of communication, theories about communication in hospitals, activities, and so on. Several categories or codes could be identified within the data recorded for any given participant, as the example indicates. The researcher works with these categories to identify the ones which are most prevalent or of greatest priority for the individual. The researcher continually compares the data collected from one participant with that of another participant in the determination of the final theme. An example of coding a participant's statement is depicted in Table 13.6.

Table 13.6 Identification of themes in a client statement	
Themes	**Select client statements:** **Experience of job loss**
loss of control betrayal unpreparedness financial stress loss of self-esteem devastation	I felt as though I was about to *explode*. I couldn't believe that *after 28 years of service to the company, of being loyal, honest, hardworking, that this could be the thanks I got. Nothing in my life prepared me for an event like this.* I always figured I would be the guy who got the gold watch and that I could retire with a *pretty good pension and a nice nest egg to fall back on.* Now, I have to *face the prospect of trying to get a job at my age* and of trying to tell my friends, neighbours and colleagues. It's *embarrassing and demeaning.* I will *never get over this ... it has ruined my life*

Source: Brockopp and Hastings-Tolsma (1995: 258)

With the advent of computer programs, data analysis has been greatly enhanced for qualitative researchers. The programs can sort, code and rearrange data in many ways.

Data analysis evaluation

The data analysis portion of a health sciences research report should be carefully scrutinised to determine whether the procedures used were appropriate and correct, and whether the findings are presented meaningfully. If this is not done, there will be no satisfactory answer to the research question. An inadequate or incorrect analysis can produce worthless or even misleading results from soundly collected data. The researcher has an intellectual and moral responsibility to assure the excellence of the data analysis. The following questions could serve as guidelines when evaluating data analysis strategies.

With regard to *scientific adequacy*:
- Does the level of measurement of the data fit with the type of statistics used?
- Is the link between the analysis and the findings logical and clear?
- Are there enough data in the form of examples, tables or graphics to allow for verification of the conclusions reached by the researcher?

Concerning *statistics*:
- Are the statistics used to describe the data the correct and most appropriate ones?
- Is the statistical result presented in clear language as well as in numerical formulation?
- Is there sufficient evidence to verify the correctness of the statistical result?

With regard to *graphics*:
- Are the graphic displays accurate, simple and clear?
- Do they make a point without the need for narrative?
- Do they enhance the quality of the argument for the conclusions reached by the researcher?

Concerning *narrative*:
- Is the method of data analysis consistent with the purpose of the study?
- Are the steps in the analysing process explicit?
- Have the research questions been answered?

Summary

In this chapter, we paid attention to data analysis strategies, dividing the statistical methods into two broad groups. We explored the descriptive techniques and discussed frequency distributions, measures of central tendency and dispersion or variability, and correlation techniques. We briefly dealt with inferential techniques and graphics. Having touched on the analysis of qualitative data, the chapter closed with a list of the general criteria for critiquing data analysis strategies.

Exercises

Complete these exercises:

1 The following scores were obtained from parents of terminally ill children who responded to a test evaluating their ability to cope with their problem: 41, 35, 38, 43, 29, 38, 27. Calculate the mean, median and mode.

2 A researcher is studying the relationship between certain employees' feelings of hopelessness and job satisfaction. She administers a job satisfaction inventory and a hopelessness inventory to 100 health care professionals and compares the results. The mean score on the hopelessness inventory is 65,8 and the mean score on the job satisfaction inventory is 72. What statistical test should she use?

3 Give an example of how standard deviation could be used in reporting an experience that you have had.

4 Rank order correlation is applied to some data and a correlation of 0,88 is found. What does this show?

5 A researcher has collected data on pulse rate and final examination marks for 10 students, and would like to know if there is a relationship between the two measures. What statistical test should he use?

6 What inferential statistic would you choose for the following sets of variables? Variable 1 is whether an amputee has a leg removed above or below the knee. Variable 2 is whether or not the amputee has shown signs of aggressive behaviour during rehabilitation.

7 Ask 10 colleagues to describe their conception of preventive health care and what it means in their daily lives. Develop a coding scheme to organise the data. What are the major themes that emerge?

14 Research reports and report evaluation

LEARNING OUTCOMES

On completion of this chapter, you should be able to demonstrate your understanding of

- research report formats
- how to correctly organise the content of a research report
- the style and ethics of report writing
- the guidelines for critiquing a research report.

Introduction

A research report is the written scientific document that a researcher produces as a result of a research study or investigation. It describes the completed study to other researchers, professionals, students or a global audience. A well-conducted and well-analysed research project is meaningless if no one hears about it. Scientific knowledge is the sum of the individual efforts of researchers working all over the world. Thus, proper communication of the researcher's results is crucial. The research report communicates information to the selected audience as clearly and accurately as possible about the research project.

The report can be viewed as the final product of the completed research process. If he/she followed and recorded the planned steps of the process, then the researcher should not find the writing of the research report difficult, as guidelines for the production of such a report are closely connected with the phases of the research process. In this chapter, we outline the purpose, format, style and organisation of a research report.

Purpose of a research report

The purpose of a research report is to convey facts and knowledge, and the findings of the research study, in a scientific, academic manner as effectively as possible. The report highlights the essence of the study and brings the study to an end. It is written in intelligible language in order for it to contribute to the scientific basis of the field of interest.

Report formats

Depending on the nature of the study, the purpose of the research and the audience of the report, there are variations in the way research reports are written and in their length.

Dissertations and theses are thorough documents, some 100-350 pages or more in length, which include exhaustive searches of the relevant literature. They are written in great detail and in a highly scientific manner. By contrast, research articles and paper presentations must show a high level of scientific quality condensed into a few pages. This means that the researcher must summarise the information about the purpose of the study, the methods used, the findings and the interpretation in a short report. Most professional journals have guidelines with regard to the format and page limit of a research article submitted for publication, while the format of a paper presentation is usually provided by the conference organiser.

The format of a report is also influenced by the intended audience. For example, a report to be presented to the average educated readership of a popular journal will present the findings in more general terms, and will avoid scientific vocabulary. It might be necessary to communicate the findings of a research study to semi-literate or illiterate people, in which case it could be done as a verbal report using audio-visual techniques such as videotapes. However, this type of report must always be supported by a written report.

Whatever the format, all research reports include a core of essential information, which we will now explore.

Sections of the report

The main sections of a research report consist of the introduction, research methodology, results, discussions and references. Added to these are the abstract, which appears at the beginning, and the appendices, which appear at the end. However, the format of a report may differ depending on the requirements of the academic institution or the journal.

The title

The title should be an accurate reflection of the research that has been performed. It must be both meaningful and brief. It should not exceed 15 words, preferably less (Talbot 1995: 631).

Abstract

The abstract must summarise the report in no more than a few short paragraphs. It must include all elements of the report. From reading the abstract, the reader should know exactly what is to follow.

Introduction to the study

Here, the research problem is introduced and the area within which the problem is situated is identified. The purpose of the study is clarified concisely and precisely. The study's significance is emphasised, and an overview of the key concepts is provided. The hypothesis, objectives or research questions are stated clearly and concisely, and logical arguments should be provided to show that each statement is plausible, reasonable and sound. Authoritative sources, including other scientists, are quoted to assess what is known about the particular issue and what remains unclear and requires further investigation. It is important that the introduction is particularly clear so that the reader grasps the precise nature of the research study and learns about its background and context.

The introduction to the study covers inter alia – the research problem, rationale for the study, significance of the study, and definitions of concepts.

Literature review

The literature review provides an overview of current knowledge of the research problem. The researcher should be able to show a grasp of the theory as well as to apply the knowledge to the research. Various theoretical viewpoints need to be taken into account. However, every aspect of the literature cannot be covered in the case of a research article or paper. Therefore, only sources relevant to the problem are cited and commented upon. The literature review maps out the main issues in the study field. In order for the researcher to keep this section concise, only the most relevant information that contributes to the argument in the study is included.

Research methodology

The purpose of this broad section is to inform the reader of how the investigation was carried out, in other words, what the researcher did to solve the research problem or to answer the research questions. It is important to remember that this section should contain enough detail to enable another researcher to replicate the investigation.

This section considers the population, sampling frame, approach and technique, sample size, data-collection method, and data processing and analysis. Here are some guidelines on ensuring that the important information is included in the report.

Subjects

A number of questions must be answered concerning the population and sample:
- Who or what was the population?
- Who were the subjects?
- How many were there?
- How were they selected?
- Why are they appropriate for this study?

Furthermore, specific information must be given concerning the population and subjects, such as their characteristics.

Instrument and data collection

The methods used to collect data form an important component of this section. A description of all tasks or types of activities that the subjects are asked to perform should be described, as well as all the material and/or instruments used. For example, if the subjects had to fill in a questionnaire, the researcher should give the main characteristics of the questionnaire; if they were tested on a certain skill with a particular instrument, the researcher must describe both the instrument and the

191

skill; if the subjects' reactions to a particular situation were observed, the researcher needs to describe in detail how this was done. He/she must also describe the considerations which led to the choice and how validity and reliability were ensured. Specially developed devices, such as questionnaires or interview schedules, should be included in an appendix.

Research design and strategy

The chosen design should be specified, including the order of succession of different activities, their duration and the instructions given to the subjects. The choices which lay behind strategy decisions should be outlined.

Data analysis

The researcher should give an account of the methods and processes that were used for analysing data. These depend on the nature of the research problem, objectives or questions, and on the type of data. If a quantitative design was used, the statistical tests applied to the obtained data should be discussed. Procedures for dealing with missing data should be explained. The presentation of validity and reliability scores is important. The reasons behind the use of specific statistical tests should be provided.

Results

This section presents the research findings. The main results following from the data analysis are presented, depending on the design and the type of analysis undertaken. If a quantitative study was done, tables, graphs and diagrams and the outcomes of statistical tests should be used to help the reader to understand the data. It is essential that these representations are used carefully, and that they have precise titles and headings so that they can be easily identified. In a quantitative study, additional information is often required, that is, the name of any statistical test used, and the value of the calculated statistic and its significance. Accuracy and conciseness must be adhered to throughout.

In a qualitative study, findings are usually presented in terms of the themes which emerged from the data and, by way of substantiation and illustration, examples of raw data will be given, for instance direct quotes from an interview transcription, or accounts of observations.

Discussion

Discussion typically incorporates the following elements:
- An interpretation and a summary of the findings, subject to validity and reliability.
- Conclusions, related to the question(s) raised in the introduction.
- Limitations identified during the study.

- Generalisation of the research findings, if applicable.
- Suggestions and recommendations.

A well-developed discussion makes sense of the research results, and must be presented in precise and concise language. Here, the researcher restates the research objectives or questions and/or hypotheses, and discusses the results with reference to these in the order that they were posed. The researcher indicates whether he/she found what was expected, and how the present results relate to existing research. Thus, the discussion should connect the findings with similar studies, and especially with the theory underlying such studies. If unexpected, inconclusive or contradictory results were obtained, possible reasons for the outcomes should be discussed.

The researcher should identify the limitations of the study and defend the validity of the findings in the light of such limitations. Limitations include factors such as the inherent weakness of the sampling method, faulty designs and controls, weaknesses in the methods used to collect data, and so forth. The researcher has the opportunity to recommend ways to minimise or eliminate the limitations of the current study, and to offer alternative methodology or improvements of the methods of the study presented. Here, too, there may be recommendations for applying the research and suggestions concerning further research.

References

The researcher must refer to the literature consulted during the study. The references should be presented in a standard manner and used consistently throughout the report. Style manuals can be consulted for information on how references should be listed. Sufficient information must be given for an interested reader to be able to identify and retrieve the sources referred to. An entry in the reference list or bibliography should feature at least the following:

- In the case of a **book**: surname(s) of the author(s) and initial(s), year of publication, title and subtitle, edition (where applicable), place of publication and publisher.
- In the case of an **article in a journal**: surname(s) of the author(s) and initial(s), year, title of the article, name of journal, volume, number of the relevant volume, page number(s).

For examples, refer to the reference list at the end of this book.

It is essential that each book and article cited in the text should appear in the reference section, with full details. Abbreviations are not allowed in bibliographies.

Style of the report

Efforts should be made to submit a clearly written report without unnecessary details and meaningless phrases.

In general, as the researcher you need to keep in mind the following points when writing a report:

- Avoid long phrases, pretentious words or complicated sentences. Short, simple sentences are far more easily understood by the reader.
- Use quotations sparingly. They should be used only when it is necessary to convey precisely the ideas of another researcher.
- Make sure that you are writing to your audience.
- Make sure that you are concise and clear. Do not introduce issues and concepts that are not strictly relevant to reporting your investigation.
- Use an objective style.
- Organise your thoughts carefully.

Technical layout of the report

Because it is a scientific document, the report must adhere to the following technical requirements, which will be governed by the specific requirements of the publisher or academic institution:

- It must have a title page that contains a title, name(s) of author(s), institutional affiliations of the authors and date (month and year) of completion.
- The pages must be numbered.
- There must be a table of contents that gives a complete list of the headings of each part of the report as well as the relevant page numbers.
- There must be a list of references to all sources used in the report.
- Headings and subheadings should be used to organise the content and make it more reader-friendly.
- Footnotes should be limited.
- The researcher must be consistent in his/her use of language tenses.
- Numbers must be written in a specific style – numbers up to ten are written in words; if the sentence begins with a figure, that figure is written as a word; and statistics such as percentages, fractions or decimal figures are expressed as numbers.

Ethics of report writing

Researchers have an obligation to the subjects who participated in the study, their colleagues and the profession to publish honest and accurate results. Attention must therefore be paid to the following ethical points:

- Data should not be invented or manipulated.
- Data or theories should not be stolen from others and reported as the researcher's.

■ The limitations and problems of carrying out the investigation should not be concealed or ignored.

■ Data should be honestly analysed and, as far as possible, interpreted without personal, political and emotional bias.

In health sciences research, ethics and honesty have widespread implications. Therefore, ethics concern not only the researcher's good intentions and appropriate treatment of the subjects, but also the issue of competence. Poorly designed and conducted research is unethical in that it may cause harm to many people.

Critical evaluation of the report

Every health care professional has the responsibility of learning to *evaluate* research, even if he/she is not a researcher. Evaluating or critiquing a research report allows the research reader to determine the merits of the study, and whether it is applicable to clinical practice or the profession. No research is perfect, particularly health sciences research, because health care professionals study people and variables in natural environments are often impossible to control.

It is important for the research reader to evaluate studies objectively, rather than emotionally (Burns & Grove 2003). Leininger (1968) has made several pertinent points about the importance of the research critique, the role of the person doing the critique and the possible reactions of the researcher whose work is critiqued. Leininger (1968: 444) defines a research critique as 'a critical estimate of a piece of research which has been carefully and systematically studied by a critic who has used specific criteria to appraise the favourable, less favourable and other general features of the research study'. The critique should be objective, constructive and advisory, and it should include the strengths, weaknesses and general features of the research being reviewed. A summary appraisal and recommendation should also be part of the critique.

Furthermore, Leininger (1968: 449) believes that the research critique is an extremely valuable and necessary means of helping any researcher to become competent in research, as well as of advancing the profession. The process of evaluating a research report requires breaking down the report into its sections and examining each section. Criteria designed to assist the evaluator in judging the relative value of each component of the research report in preceding chapters follows.

When undertaking a critique, the evaluator *should*

■ be objective

■ identify positive aspects of the study and use positive terms wherever possible

■ consider the report in a balanced way, that is, identify inadequacies as well as adequacies

195

■ make comments specific to the work being reviewed and provide explanation, where necessary

■ discuss strengths first, followed by weaknesses.

When undertaking a critique, the evaluator *should not*
■ search dogmatically for mistakes
■ be petty
■ use terms such as 'bad', 'good' and 'nice', as they are meaningless in this context.

Common errors that the evaluator can look out for in the report are as follows:
■ Insufficient or inadequate information may be provided in one or more components of the research process.
■ Theoretical or conceptual frameworks may not fit or make sense; in other words, they are illogical.
■ Sentences, paragraphs or parts may be confusing, which usually means that they have been expressed poorly.
■ Components may be more complicated than necessary, as is the case when the researcher tries to combine too many theories or to put too much into a design.
■ Information may be inappropriate, inapplicable or unrelated to the research question or other parts of the study.
■ Statements may be questionable, or supported by insufficient data or other evidence.

The first-time evaluator will understandably find critiquing difficult to do. It takes time and practice to develop competence. It is unrealistic for an evaluator to be skilled without practice, and delivering constructive criticism is a valuable skill.

Summary

In this chapter, we outlined the general format that a researcher must follow when writing up his/her study results. We emphasised the responsibility that he/she has to use a clear, comprehensive and accurate style to facilitate the readers' understanding or so that other researchers could replicate the project. The researcher is also ethically bound, we pointed out, to report the findings in an unbiased and truthful manner. Lastly, we explored aspects of the critical evaluation of a research report.

Exercises

Complete these exercises:

1 Select two or three articles from research journals. Identify the key elements of each report.

2 Select another research article from a research journal and evaluate it, using the criteria we outline in this chapter.

3 Comment on the following statements:

   a) 'Novice researchers have few skills or experiences which qualify them to critique research.'

   b) 'If critics do not find as many positive features in their evaluation as they find negative features, they are being overly critical.'

4 In the section of the report entitled 'Research design and strategy', what elements of research does the writer inform the readers about?

5 Identify a journal in which you could present a report.

6 Read the guidelines to authors.

Glossary

abstracts (research abstracts). Brief summaries of research studies; generally contain the purpose, methods, and major findings of the study. It usually precedes the study report.

accessible population. The group of people or objects that is available to the researcher for a particular study.

adequacy. A desirable attribute of sampling whereby sufficient numbers of subjects (or objects) have been sampled to represent the population accurately.

acquiescence response set. A type of response set bias in which a subject may have a tendency to answer 'yes' or agree with the content of the questions.

ambiguous questions. Questions that contain words that may be interpreted in more that one way.

anonymity. The identity of research subjects is unknown, even to the study investigator.

applied research. Research that is conducted to find a solution to an immediate, practical problem.

assumptions. Basic ideas that are held to be true but have not necessarily been proven; assumptions may be explicit or implicit.

attitude scales. Self-report data collection instruments that ask respondents to report their attitudes or feelings on a continuum.

attribute variables. See demographic variables.

bar graph. A figure used to represent a frequency distribution of nominal or ordinal data.

basic research (pure research). Research that is conducted to generate knowledge rather than solve immediate problems.

bias. Any influence that produces a distortion in the results of a study or that strongly favours the outcome of a particular finding of a research study.

bimodal. A frequency distribution that contains two identical high-frequency values.

bracketing. In qualitative data analysis, the process of putting aside what is known about a study topic to allow the data to convey undistorted information.

bivariate study. A research study in which the relationship between two variables is examined.

cells. Boxes in a table that are formed by the intersection of rows and columns.

chi-square test (X^2). A non-parametric statistical test that is used to compare sets of data that are in the form of frequencies or percentages (nominal level data).

class interval. A group of scores in a frequency distribution.

clinical research. Clinical research studies involving clients or study alternatives.

closed-ended questions. Questions that require respondents to choose from given alternatives.

cluster random sampling. A random sampling process that involves two or more stages. The population is first listed by clusters or categories (e.g. hospitals) and then the sample elements (e.g. hospital administrators) are randomly selected from these clusters.

cohort study. A special type of longitudinal study in which subjects are studied who have been born during one particular period or who have similar backgrounds

collectively exhaustive categories. Categories are provided for every possible answer.

columns. Vertical entries in a table.

comparative studies. Studies in which intact groups are compared on some dependent variable. The researcher is not able to manipulate the independent variable, which is frequently some inherent characteristics of the subjects, such as age or educational level.

comparison group. A group of subjects in an experimental study that does not receive any experimental treatment or receives an alternate treatment such as the 'normal' or routine treatment.

computer-assisted literature searches. The use of a computer to obtain bibliographic references that have been stored in a database.

concept. A word picture or mental idea stored in a database.

conceptual framework. A background or information for a study; a less well-developed structure than a theoretical framework. Concepts are related in a logical manner by the researcher.

conceptual model. Symbolic presentation of concepts and the relationships between these concepts.

concurrent validity. A type of criterion validity of an instrument in which a determination is made of the instrument's ability to obtain a measurement of subjects' behaviour that is comparable to some other criterion used to indicate that behaviour.

confidence interval. A range of values that, with a specified degree of probability, is thought to contain the population value.

confidentiality. The identity of the research subjects is known only to the study investigator (s).

construct. A highly abstract phenomenon that cannot be directly observed but must be inferred by certain concrete or less abstract indicators of the phenomenon.

construct validity. The ability of an instrument to measure the construct that it is intended to measure.

content analysis. A data-analysis method that examines communication messages that are usually in written form.

content validity. The degree to which an instrument covers the scope and range of information that is sought.

contingency table. A table that visually displays the relationship between sets of nominal data.

control group. A group of subjects in an experimental study that does not receive the experimental treatment (see *comparison group*).

convenience sampling (accidental samplings). A non-probability sampling procedure that involves the selection of the most readily available people or objects for a study.

correlation. The extent to which values of one variable (X) are related to the values of a second variable (Y). Correlations can be either positive or negative.

correlation coefficient. A statistic that represents the magnitude and direction of a relationship between two variables. Correlation coefficients range from -1.00 (perfect negative relationship) to + 1.00 (perfect positive relationship).

correlation studies. Research studies that examine the strength relationships between variables.

correlation validity. The extent to which an instrument corresponds or correlates with some criterion measure of the information that is being sought; the ability of an instrument to determine subjects' responses at present or predict subjects' responses in the future.

critical region (region of rejection). An area in a theoretical sampling distribution that contains the critical values, or values that are considered to be statistically significant.

critical value. A scientific cut-off point that denotes the value in a theoretical distribution at which all obtained values from a sample that are equal to or beyond that point are said to be statistically significant.

critique. Analytical examination of a research report or proposal that involves a systematic assessment based on accepted standards of inquiry and communication.

cross-sectional study. A research study that collects data on subjects at one point in time.

data. The pieces of information or facts collected during a research study.

deductive reasoning. A reasoning process that proceeds from the general to the specific, from theory to empirical data.

degrees of freedom (df). A concept in inferential statistics that concerns the number of values that are free to vary.

Delphi technique. A data-collection method that uses several rounds of questions to seek a consensus on a particular topic from a group of experts on the topic.

demographic questions. Questions that gather data on characteristics of the subjects (see *demographic variables*).

demographic variables. Subject characteristics such as age, educational levels and marital status.

dependent variable. The 'effect'; the variable that is influenced by the independent variable.

descriptive statistics. That group of statistics that organises and summarises numerical data obtained from populations and samples.

descriptive studies. Research studies in which phenomena are described or the relationship between variables is examined; no attempt is made to determine cause-and -effect relationships.

double-barrelled questions. Questions that ask two questions in one.

element. A single member of a population.

empirical data. Objective data gathered through the sense organs.

empirical generalisation. A summary statement about the occurrence of phenomena that is based on empirical data from a number of different research studies.

equivalence reliability. The degree to which two forms of an instrument obtain the same results or two or more observers obtain the same results when using a single instrument to measure a variable.

ethnographic studies. Research studies that involve the collection and analysis of date about cultural groups.

evidence-based practice. The integration of best research evidence with clinical expertise and patient values.

experimenter effect. A threat to the internal validity of a research study that occurs when the researcher's behaviour influences the subjects' behaviour in a way that is not intended by the researcher.

explanatory studies. Research studies that are conducted when little is known about the phenomenon that is being studied.

ex post facto **studies.** Studies in which the variation on the dependent variable has already occurred in the past, and the researcher, 'after the fact', is trying to determine if the variation that has occurred in the independent variable has any influence on the dependent variable that is being measured in the present.

external criticism (external appraisal, external examination). A type of examination of historical data that is concerned with the authenticity or genuineness of the data. External criticism would be used to determine if a letter was actually written by the person whose signature was contained on the letter.

external validity. The degree to which study results can be generalised to other people and other research settings.

extraneous variable. A type of variable that is not the variable of interest to a researcher but that may influence the results of a study. Other terms for extraneous variable are intervening variable and confounding variable.

face validity. A subjective determination that an instrument is adequate for obtaining the desired information; on the surface of the 'face' of the instrument it appears to be an adequate means of obtaining the desired data.

field studies. Research studies that are conducted 'in the field' or in a real-life setting.

filler questions. Questions used to distract respondents from the purpose of other questions that are being asked.

frequency counts. The listing or counting of each observation in a category; appropriate for nominal and ordinal data.

frequency polygon. A graph that uses dots connected with straight lines to represent the frequency distribution of interval or ratio data. A dot is placed above the midpoint of each class interval.

grounded theory studies. Research studies in which data are collected and analysed and then a theory is developed that is 'grounded' in the data.

Hawthorne effect. A threat to the internal validity of a research study that occurs when study participants respond in a certain manner because they are aware that they are involved in a research study.

health sciences research. A systematic, objective process of analysing phenomena of importance to health scientists.

histogram. A graph used to represent the frequency distribution of variables measured at the interval or ratio level.

historical studies. Research studies that are concerned with the identification, location, evaluation, and synthesis of data from the past.

history. A threat to the internal validity of an experimental research study; some event besides the experimental treatment occurs between the pre-treatment and post-treatment measurement of the dependent variable, and this event influences the dependent variable.

hypothesis. A statement of the predicted relationship between two or more variables.

independent variable. The cause or the variable that is sought to influence the dependent variable; in experimental research it is the variable that is manipulated by the researcher.

indexes. Compilations of reference materials that provide information on books and periodicals.

inductive reasoning. A reasoning process that proceeds from the specific to the general, from empirical data to theory.

inferential statistics. The group of statistics that is concerned with the characteristics of populations and that uses sample data to make an inference about the population.

informed consent. A subject voluntarily agrees to participate in a research study in which he or she has full understanding of the study before the study begins.

interaction effect. The result of two variables acting in conjunction.

internal criticism. A type of examination of historical data that is concerned with the accuracy of the data. Internal criticism would be used to determine if a document contained an accurate recording of events as they actually happened.

internal validity. The degree to which changes in the dependent variable (effect) can be attributed to the independent or experimental variable (cause).

Interobserver reliability. See *interrater reliability*.

interrater reliability (interobserver reliability). The degree to which two or more independent judges are in agreement about ratings or observations of events or behaviours.

interval level of measurement. Data can be categorised and ranked, and the distance between the ranks can be specified. There is no absolute zero level. Temperature readings are examples of interval data.

interview. A method of data collection in which the interviewer obtains responses from a subject in a face-to-face encounter or through a telephone call.

interview schedule. An instrument containing a set of questions, directions for asking those questions, and space to record the respondents' answers.

laboratory studies. Research studies in which subjects are studied in a special environment that has been created and controlled by the researcher.

Likert scale. An attitude scale named after its developer, Renis Likert. These scales usually contain five or seven responses for each item, ranging from 'strongly agree' to 'strongly disagree'.

limitations. Weaknesses in a study; uncontrolled variables.

longitudinal study. Subjects are followed during a period in the future and data are collected at two or more time periods.

manipulation. The independent or experimental variable is controlled by the researcher to determine its effect on the dependent variable.

maturation. A threat to the internal validity of an experimental research study that occurs when changes take place within study subjects as a result of the passage of time (growing older, taller) and these changes may affect the study results.

methodological studies. Research studies that are concerned with the development, testing and evaluation of research instruments and methods.

mortality. A threat to the internal validity of an experimental research study that occurs when subject drop-out rate is different between the experimental group and the comparison group.

multimodal. A frequency distribution in which more than two values have the same high frequency.

mutual exclusive categories. Categories are uniquely distinct; no overlap occurs between categories.

negative relationship (inverse relationship). A relationship between two variables in which there is a tendency for the values of one variable to increase as the values of the other variable decrease.

negatively skewed. A frequency distribution in which the tail of the distribution points to the left.

nominal level of measurement. The lowest level of measurement; data are 'named' or categorised, such as race and marital status.

non-directional research hypothesis. A type of research hypothesis in which a prediction is made that a relationship exists between variables, but the type of relationship is not specified.

non-equivalent control group design. A type of quasi-experimental design, similar to the pre-test-post-test control group experimental design, with the exception of random assignment of subjects to groups.

non-parametric tests (distribution-free statistics). A type of inferential statistics that is not concerned with population parameters; requirements for their use are less stringent and they can be used with nominal and ordinal data and small sample sizes.

non-participant observer-overt. Research observer openly states that she or he is conducting research and provides subjects with information about the type of data that will be collected.

non-probability sampling. A sampling process in which a sample is selected from elements or members of a population through non-random methods; includes convenience, quota, and purposive.

non-symmetrical distribution (skewed distribution). Frequency distribution in which the distribution has an off-center peak. If the tail of the distribution points to the right, the distribution is said to be positively skewed, if the tail of the distribution points to the left, the distribution is said to be negatively skewed.

normal curve. A bell-shaped curve that graphically depicts a normally distributed frequency distribution (see *normal distribution*).

normal distribution. A symmetrical, bell-shaped theoretical distribution; has one central peak or set of values in the middle of the distribution.

null hypothesis (HO). A statistical hypothesis that predicts that no relationship exists between variables; the hypothesis that is subjected to statistical analysis.

observational research. A data-collection method in which data are collected through visual observations.

open-ended questions. Questions that allow respondents to answer in their own words.

operational definition. The definition of a variable that identifies how the variable will be observed or measured.

ordinal level of measurement. Data can be categorised and placed in order; small, medium, and large is an example of a set of ordinal data.

parameter. A numerical characteristic of a population; e.g. the average educational level of people living in Gauteng province.

parametric tests. A type of inferential statistic that is concerned with population parameters. When parametric tests are used assumptions are made that (a) the level of measurement of the data is interval or ratio, (b) data are taken from the populations that are normally distributed on the variable that is being measured, and (c) data are taken from populations that have equal variances on the variable that is being measured.

participant observer – covert. Research observer interacts with the subjects and observes their behaviour without their knowledge.

participant observer – overt. Research observer interacts with subjects openly and with the full awareness of those people who will be observed.

percentage (%). A statistic that represents the proportion of a subgroup to a total group, expressed as a percentage ranging from 0 to 100 percent.

percentile. A data point below which lies a certain percentage of the values in a frequency distribution.

personality inventories. Self-report measures used to assess the differences through the descriptions of the meanings of these experiences provided by the people involved.

pilot study. A small-scale, trial run of an actual research study.

population. A complete set of persons or objects that possess some common characteristic that is of interest to the researcher.

positively skewed. A frequency distribution in which the tail of the distribution points to the right.

positive relationship (direct relationship). A relationship between two variables in which the variables tend to vary together; as the values of one variable increase, the values of the other variable increase.

predictive validity. A type of criterion validity of an instrument in which a determination is made of the instrument's ability to predict the behaviour of subjects in the future.

pre-existing data. Existing information that has not been collected for research purposes.

pre-experimental design. A type of experimental design in which the researcher has little control over the research situation; includes the one-shot case study and the one-group pre-test/post-test design.

primary source. An account of research study that is presented by the original researcher(s); in historical data, primary sources are those that provide first-hand information or direct evidence of an event.

probability sampling. The use of a random sampling procedure to select a sample from elements or members of a population; includes simple, stratified, cluster, and systematic random sampling techniques.

probes. Prompting questions that encourage the respondent to elaborate on the topic that is being discussed.

projective technique. Self-report measure in which a subject is asked to respond to stimuli that are designed to be ambiguous or to have no definite meaning. The responses reflect the internal feelings of the subject that are projected upon the external stimuli.

proposal. A plan or suggestion, especially a formal or written one, put forward for consideration or discussion by others.

reliability. The consistency and dependability of a research instrument to measure a variable; types of reliability are stability, equivalence, and internal consistency.

replication study. A research study that repeats or duplicates an earlier research study, with all the essential elements of the original study held intact. A different sample or setting may be used.

research design. The overall plan for gathering data in a research study.

research hypothesis (H1). An alternative hypothesis to the statistical null hypothesis; predicts the researcher's actual expectations about the outcome of a study; also called scientific, substantive, and theoretical.

research instruments (research tools). Devices used to collect data in research studies.

research report. A written or oral summary of a research study.

retrospective studies. Studies in which the dependent variable is identified in the present (e.g. a disease condition) and an attempt is made to determine the independent variable (e.g. cause of the disease) that occurred in the past.

rows. Horizontal entries in a table.

sample. A subset of the population that is selected to represent the population.

sampling bias. (1) The difference between sample data and population data that can be attributed to a faulty selection process; (2) a threat to the external validity of a research study that occurs when subjects are not randomly selected from the population.

sampling distribution. A theoretical frequency distribution that is based on an infinite number of samples. Sampling distributions are based on mathematical formulas and logic.

sampling error. Random fluctuations in data that occur when a sample is selected to represent a population.

sampling frame. A listing of all the elements of the population from which a sample is to be chosen.

scatter plot (scatter diagram, scattergram). A graphic presentation of the relationship between two variables. The graph contains variables plotted on an X axis and a Y axis. Pairs of scores are plotted by the placement of dots to indicate where each pair of X's and Y's intersect.

secondary sources. In the research literature, it is an account of a research study that is written by someone other than the study investigators; in historical data, secondary sources and secondhand information or data provided by someone who did not observe the event.

selection bias. A threat to the internal validity of an experimental research study that occurs when study results are attributed to the experimental treatment when, in fact, the results may be due to pretreatment differences between the subjects in the experimental and comparison groups.

semantic differential. Attitude scale that asks subjects to indicate their position or attitude about some concept along continuum between two adjectives or phrases that are presented in relation to the concept that is being measured.

skew. A frequency distribution that is non-symmetrical

snowball sampling. A sampling methods that involves the assistance of study subjects to help obtain other potential subjects.

standard deviation (SD). A measure of variability; the statistic that indicates the average deviation or variation of all the values in a set of data from the mean value of that data.

standard error of the mean (sx). The standard deviation of the sampling distribution of the mean.

structured interviews. The interviews ask the same questions in the same manner of all respondents.

survey studies. Research studies in which self-report data are collected from a sample in order to determine the characteristics of a population.

symmetrical distributions. Frequency distributions in which both halves of the distribution are the same.

theoretical framework. A study framework based on prepositional statements from a theory of theories.

theory. A set of related statements that describes or explains phenomena in a systematic way.

time sampling. Observations of events or behaviours that are made during certain specified time periods.

triangulation. The use of multiple methods or perspectives to collect and interpret data about some phenomenon; to converge on an accurate representation of reality.

univariate study. A research study in which only one variable is examined.

unstructured interviews. The interviewer is given a great deal of freedom to direct the course of the interview; the interviewer's main goal is to encourage the respondent to talk freely about the topic that is being explored.

unstructured observations. The researcher describes behaviours as they are viewed, with no preconceived ideas of what will be seen.

validity. The ability of an instrument to measure the variable that it is intended to measure.

variable. A characteristic or attribute of a person or object that differs among the persons or objects that are being studied, e.g. age, blood type.

volunteers. Subjects who have offered to participate in a study.

Bibliography

Aber, C & Hawkins, J. 1992. Portrayal of nurses in advertisements in medical and nursing journals. *Image: Journal of Nursing Scholarship* 24(4), 289–93.

Ader, HJ & Mellenbergh, GJ. 1999. *Research Methodology in the Social, Behavioural and Life Sciences.* London: Sage.

Ahrens, EH. 1992. *The Crisis in Clinical Research.* New York: Oxford University Press.

Alien, JD. 1989. Women who successfully manage their weight. *Western Journal of Nursing Research* 11(6), 657–75.

Altman, DG. n.d. *Statistics and Ethics in Medical Research.* Harrow, Middlesex: Clinical Research Centre.

Anderson, JM. 1991. Immigrant women speak of chronic illness: The social construction of the devalued self. *Journal of Advanced Nursing* 16(6), 710–11.

Arminger, B. 1977. Ethics of nursing research: Profile, principles, perspective. *Nursing Research* 26(5), 330–36.

Babbie, E & Mouton, J. 2001. *The Practice of Social Research.* Cape Town: Oxford University Press.

Banonis, BC. 1989. The lived experience of recovering from addiction: A phenomenological study. *Nursing Science Quarterly* 2(1), 37–43.

Bless, C & Higson-Smith, C. 2000. *Fundamentals of Social Research Methods: An African Perspective,* 3 ed. Cape Town: Juta.

Bond, M. 1980. Shave it ... or save it? *Nursing Times* 76(9), 362–63.

Booysen, S. 2003. Designing a questionnaire. In *Intellectual Tools – Skills for the Human Sciences,* 2 ed, ed D Rossouw. Pretoria: Van Schaik.

Botes, A. 1992. 'n Model vir kwalitatiewe navorsing in die verpleegkunde. *Curationis* 15(4), 36–42.

Breakwell, GM, Hammond, S & Fife-Schaw, C. 2000. *Research Methods in Psychology,* 2 ed. London: Sage.

Brink, JJ & Wood, MJ. 1994. *Basic Steps in Planning Nursing Research,* 4 ed. Boston: Jones and Bartlett.

Brink, PJ & Wood, MJ. 1998. *Advanced Design in Nursing Research,* 2 ed. London: Sage.

Brink, P & Wood, MJ. 1999. *Basic Steps in Planning Nursing Research.* Boston: Jones and Bartlett.

Brockopp, DY & Hastings-Tolsma, MX. 1995. *Fundamentals of Nursing Research.* Boston: Jones and Bartlett.

Brown, B, Crawford, P & Hicks, C. 2003. *Evidence-based Research: Dilemmas and Debates in Health Care.* Berkshire: Open University Press.

Burns, N & Grove, SK. 2003. *Understanding Nursing Research,* 3 ed. Philadelphia: Saunders.

Burns, N & Grove, SK. 2005. *The Practice of Nursing Research,* 5 ed. Philadelphia: Elsevier.

Bush, CT. 1985. *Nursing Research.* Reston, VA: Reston Publishers.

Bush, H. 1979. Models for nursing. *Advances in Nursing Science* 1(2), 13–21.

Campbell, D & Stanley, J. 1966. *Experimental and Quasi-experimental Designs for Research.* Chicago: Rand McNally.

Carper, BA. 1978. Fundamental patterns of knowing in nursing. *Advances in Nursing Science* 1(1), 13–23.

Chenitz, WC & Swanson, JM. 1986. *From Practice to Grounded Theory: Qualitative Research in Nursing.* Menlo Park, California: Addison-Wesley.

Chinn, PL & Kramer, MK. 1991. *Theory and Nursing: A Systematic Approach.* St Louis: Mosby.

Christiansen, CH. 1981. Editorial: Toward resolution of a crisis: Research requisites in occupational therapy. *The Occupational Therapy Journal of Research* 1, 116–24.

Clare, J & Hamilton, H. 2003. *Writing Research: Transforming Data into Text.* Edinburgh: Churchill Livingstone.

Clifford, CL & Clark, J (eds.). 2004. *Getting Research into Practice.* Edinburgh: Churchill Livingstone.

Cohen, J. 1977. *Statistical Power Analysis for the Behavioural Sciences.* New York: Academic Press.

Collaizi, PF. 1978. Psychological research as the phenomenologist views it. In *Existential Phenomenological Alternatives for Psychology,* ed R Valle & M King. New York: Oxford University Press.

Cook, C & Campbell, D. 1979. *Quasi-experimentation: Design and Analysis Issues for Field Settings.* Chicago: Rand McNally.

Corbin, J & Strauss, A. 1990. Grounded theory research: Procedures, canons and evaluative criteria. *Qualitative Sociology* 13(1), 3–21.

Cormack, DPS. 1991. *The Research Process in Nursing,* 2 ed. Oxford: Blackwell Science.

Cummings, SE, Dean, R & Newell, D. 1960. Disengagement: A tentative theory of aging. *Sociometry* 23(1), 23–35.

De Vos, AS (ed). 2002. *Research at Grass Roots,* 2 ed. Pretoria: Van Schaik.

Declaration of Helsinki. 1986. In *Philosophical Medical Ethics,* R Gillan. Chichester: Wiley.

Denzin, NK. 1989. *Interpretive Interactionism.* Newbury Park, California: Sage.

Dickhoff, J & James, P. 1968. A theory of theories: A position paper. *Nursing Research* 17(3), 197–203.

Dowd, TT. 1991. Discovering older women's experience of urinary incontinence. *Research in Nursing and Health* 14, 179–86.

Du Plooy, GM. 2001. *Communication Research: Techniques, Methods and Applications.* Lansdowne: Juta.

Dubin, R. 1978. *Theory Building,* rev ed. New York: Free Press.

Fawcett, J & Downs, F. 1986. *The Relationship of Theory and Research.* Norwalk, Connecticut: Appleton-Century-Crofts.

Fawcett, J. 1983. Hallmarks of success in nursing theory development. In *Advances in Nursing Theory Development,* ed PL Chinn, 3–17. Rockville, Maryland: Aspen.

Fawcett, J. 1989. *Analysis and Evaluation of Conceptual Models of Nursing.* Philadelphia: Aspen.

Feyerabend, P. 1975. *Against Method.* London: Verso.

Field, PA & Morse, JM. 1985. *Nursing Research: The Application of Qualitative Approaches.* Kent: Croome Helm.

Flaskerud, J & Holloran, E. 1980. Areas of agreement in nursing theory development. *Advances in Nursing Science* 3(1), 1–7.

Ganong, L, Coleman, M & Riley, C. 1988. Health care sciences students' stereotypes of married and unmarried pregnant clients. *Research in Health Care Sciences and Health* 11, 333–42.

Garbers, JG (ed). 1996. *Effective Research in the Human Sciences.* Pretoria: Van Schaik.

Giorgi, A. 1970. *Psychology as a Human Science.* New York: Harper and Row.

Giovanetti, P. 1981. Sampling techniques. In *Research Methodology and its Application to Nursing*, ed YM Williamson, 169–90. New York: Wiley.

Glaser, B & Strauss, A. 1967. *The Discovery of Grounded Theory: Strategies for Qualitative Research.* Chicago: Aldine.

Guba, EY. 1990. *The Paradigm Dialogue.* Newbury Park: Sage.

Hastings, J (ed). 1961. *Encyclopedia of Religion and Ethics.* New York: Scribner.

Havighurst, R. 1968. Personality and patterns of aging. *The Gerontologist* 8(1), 20–30.

Hinds, PS, Scandrett-Hibden, S & McAulay, LS. 1990. Further assessment of a method to estimate reliability and validity of qualitative research findings. *Journal of Advanced Nursing* 15(4), 430–35.

Hockey, L. 1991. The nature and purpose of research. In *The Research Process in Health Care Sciences*, ed DPS Cormack. London: Blackwell Science.

Human Sciences Research Council n.d. Research Code. Pretoria: HSRC.

Hutchison, J. 1977. *Living Options in World Philosophy.* Honolulu: University Press of Hawaii.

Jones, PS & Martinson, IM. 1992. The experience of bereavement in caregivers of family members with Alzheimer's disease. *Image, Journal of Nursing Scholarship* 24(3), 172–76.

Kayser-Jones, J, Davis, A, Wiener, CC & Higgins, SS. 1990. An ethical analysis of an elder's treatment. *Nursing Outlook* 37(6), 267–70.

Keller, C. 1991. Seeking normalcy: The experience of coronary artery by-pass surgery. *Research in Nursing and Health* 14(4), 173–78.

King, IM. 1981. *A Theory for Nursing Systems, Concepts, Process.* New York: Wiley.

Kinzel, D. 1991. Self-identified health concerns of two homeless groups. *Western Journal of Nursing Research* 13, 181–90.

Kirk, J & Miller, ML. 1986. *Reliability and Validity in Qualitative Research.* Beverley Hills: Sage.

Kuhn, TS. 1970. *The Structure of Scientific Revolutions*, 2 ed. Chicago: University of Chicago Press.

Kuhn, TS. 1977. Second thoughts on paradigms. In *The Structure of Scientific Theory*, ed F Suppe, 459–82. Urbana: University of Illinois Press.

Lancaster, W & Lancaster, J. 1981. Models and model building in nursing. *Advances in Nursing Science* 3(3), 31–42.

Landau, L. 1977. *Progress and its Problems. Toward a Theory of Scientific Growth.* Berkeley: University of California.

Le Compte, MD & Goetz, JP. 1982. Problems of reliability and validity in ethnographic research. *Review of Educational Research* 52(1), 31–60.

Leedy, PD. 1993. *Practical Research: Planning and Design.* New York: Macmillan.

Leininger, MM. 1968. The research critique: Nature, function and act. *Nursing Research* 17(5), 444–49.

Leininger, MM (ed). 1985. *Qualitative Research Methods in Nursing.* Orlando: Grune & Gratton.

Leininger, MM. 1991. *Culture Care, Diversity and Universality. A Theory of Nursing*. New York: NLN.

Lincoln, Y & Guba, E. 1985. *Naturalistic Enquiry*. Beverley Hills, California: Sage.

LoBiondo-Wood, G & Haber, J. 1990. *Nursing Research: Methods, Critical Appraisal and Utilisation*. St Louis: Mosby.

Luyas, GT. 1991. An explanatory model of diabetes. *Western Journal of Nursing Research* 13, 181–90.

Marriner, A. 1986. *Nursing Theorists and their Work*. St Louis: Mosby.

Masterman, M. 1970. The nature of a paradigm. In *Criticism and the Growth of Knowledge*, eds I Lakatos and A Musgrave. Cambridge: Cambridge University Press.

Meleis, A. 1985. *Theoretical Nursing: Development and Progress*. Philadelphia: Lippincott.

Merton, R. 1968. *Social Theory and Social Structure*. New York: Free Press.

Miles, MB & Huberman, AM. 1984. *Qualitative Data Analysis: A Source Book of New Methods*. Newbury Park: Sage.

Miles, MG & Huberman, AM. 1994. *Qualitative Data Analysis: A Sourcebook of New Methods*. Beverley Hills, California: Sage.

Moccia, P. 1986. New approaches to theory development. (Pub no 15-1992). New York: National League for Nursing.

Moody, L, Vera, H, Blanks, C & Visscher, M. 1989. Developing questions of substance for nursing science. *Western Journal of Nursing Research* II, 392–403.

Moody, LE. 1990. *Advancing Nursing Science through Research* I. Newbury Park: Sage.

Morse, JM (ed). 1992. *Qualitative Health Research*. Newbury Park: Sage.

Mouton, J. 1996. *Understanding Social Research*. Pretoria: Van Schaik.

Mouton, J & Marais, HC. 1988. *Basic Concepts in the Methodology of the Social Sciences*. Pretoria: HSRC.

Muir Gray, JA. 1997. *Evidence-based Health Care: How to make Health Policy and Management Decisions*. New York: Churchill Livingstone.

Munhall, PL. 2001. *Nursing Research – A Qualitative Perspective*, 3 ed. Boston: Jones and Bartlett.

Munhall, PL & Oiler, CJ (eds). 1986. *Nursing Research: A Qualitative Perspective*. Connecticut: Appleton-Century-Crofts.

Neuman, B. 1989. *The Neuman Systems Model*, 2 ed. Norwalk, Connecticut: Appleton & Lange.

Newman, M. 1983. *Theory Development in Nursing*. Philadelphia: Davis.

Neuman, WL. 2000. *Social Research Methods: Qualitative and Quantitative Approaches*, 4 ed. Boston: Allyn & Bacon.

Nieswiadomy, R. 1993. *Foundations of Nursing Research*. Norwalk, Connecticut: Appleton & Lange.

Nuremberg Code. In *Nursing Ethics through the Lifespan*, FL Bandman & B Bandman. 1990. Norwalk, Connecticut: Appleton & Lange.

Orem, D. 1985. *Concepts of Practice*, 3 ed. New York: McGraw-Hill.

Ornery, A. 1988. Ethnography. In *Paths to Knowledge*, ed B Sarter. New York: NLN.

Ottenbacher, K. 1990. Editorial: Occupational therapy curricula and practice: Skill based or knowledge based. *The Occupational Therapy Journal of Research* 10(1), 7–11.

Owen, BD. 1989. The magnitude of low-back problem in nursing. *Western Journal of Nursing Research* 11(2), 234–42.

Palmer, I. 1977. Florence Nightingale: Reformer, reactionary, researcher. *Nursing Research* 26(2), 84–89.

Parse, RR. 1987. *Nursing Science: Major Paradigms, Theories and Critiques.* Philadelphia: WB Saunders.

Phillips, LR. 1986. *A Clinician's Guide to the Critique and Utilisation of Nursing Research.* Norwalk, Connecticut: Appleton-Century-Crofts.

Polgar, S & Thomas, SA. 2000. *Introduction to Research in the Health Sciences,* 4 ed. Edinburgh: Churchill Livingstone.

Polit, DF & Hungler, BP. 1991. *Nursing Research: Principles and Methods.* Philadelphia: Lippincott.

Polit, DF & Hungler, BP. 1993. *Essentials of Nursing Research.* Philadelphia: Lippincott.

Polit, DF & Hungler, BP. 1995. *Nursing Research: Principles and Methods,* 6 ed. Philadelphia: Lippincott.

Polit, DF, Beck CT & Hungler, BP. 2001. *Essentials of Nursing Research: Methods, Appraisal, and Utilization,* 5 ed. Philadelphia: Lippincott.

Proctor, S & Renfrew, M (eds.). 2001. *Linking Research and Practice in Midwifery: A Guide to Evidence-based Practice.* Edinburgh: Baillière Tindall.

Readers Digest Oxford Complete Wordfinder. 1993. Oxford University Press.

Reid, N. 1993. *Nursing Research by Degrees.* Oxford: Blackwell Science.

Riemen, DJ. 1986. The essential structure of a caring interaction: Doing phenomenology. In *Nursing Research: A Qualitative Perspective,* eds PL Munhall & CJ Oiler. Norwalk, Connecticut: Appleton-Century-Crofts.

Roberts, CA & Burke, SO. 1989. *Nursing Research: A Quantitative and Qualitative Approach.* Boston: Jones and Bartlett.

Rogers, ME. 1970. *An Introduction to the Theoretical Basis of Nursing.* Philadelphia: FA Davis.

Romney, ML. 1980. Pre-delivery shaving: An unjustified thought. *Journal of Obstetrics and Gynaecology* 1(1), 33.

Rose, JE. 1990. Psychological health of women: A phenomenological study of women's inner strength. *Advances in Nursing Science* 7(1), 13–18.

Rossouw, D (ed). 2003. *Intellectual Tools: Skills for the Human Sciences,* 2 ed. Pretoria: Van Schaik.

Roy, C. 1984. *Introduction to Nursing: An Adaptation Model,* 2 ed. Englewood Cliffs, New Jersey: Prentice-Hall.

Russell, B. 1945. *A History of Western Philosophy.* New York: Simon & Schuster.

Ruth, MV & White, CM. 1981. Data collection: Sample. In *Reading for Nursing Research,* eds SD Krampitz & N Pavlovich, 93–97. St Louis: Mosby.

Sackett, DL, Strauss, SE, Richardson, WS, Rosenberg & Haynes 2000. *Evidence-based Medicine,* 2 ed. Edinburgh: Churchill Livingstone.

Santopinto, MDA. 1989. The relentless drive to be ever thinner: A study using the phenomenological method. *Nursing Science Quarterly* 2(1), 18–28.

Seaman, CHC. 1987. *Research Methods: Principles, Practice and Theory for Nursing*. Norwalk, Connecticut: Appleton & Lange.

Searle, C. 1990. Research as a modifier of the constraints in developing nursing practice in South Africa: An overview. In *Nursing Research for Nursing Practice: An International Perspective*, ed R Begman. London: Chapman & Hall.

Selltiz, C, Wrightsman, LC & Cook, WS. 1976. *Research Methods in Social Relations*, 3 ed. New York: Holt, Rinehart & Winston.

Sharrock, W. 1979. Portraying the professional relationship. In *Health Education in Practice*, ed DC Anderson. London: Croome Helm.

Shelley, SJ. 1984. *Research Methods in Nursing and Health*. Boston: Little Brown.

Simmons, LW & Henderson, V. 1964. *Nursing Research: A Survey and Assessment*. New York: Appleton-Century-Crofts.

Smith, JA. 1981. The idea of health: A philosophic inquiry. *Advances in Nursing Science* 3(3), 43–50.

Sophier, R. 1993. Filial reconstruction: A theory of development through adversity. *Qualitative Health Research* 3, 465–92.

South African Medical Research Council. 1987. Ethical Considerations in Medical Research.

South African Nursing Association. 1990. Ethical Standards for Nursing Research. Pretoria: SANA.

Spiegelberg, H. 1976. *The Phenomenological Movements* I (II). The Hague: Martinus Nijhoff.

Spradley, J. 1980. *Participant Observation*. New York: Holt, Rinehart & Winston.

Stake, RE. 2003. Case studies. In *Strategies of Qualitative Inquiry*, 2 ed, eds NK Denzin & YS Lincoln. Thousand Oakes: Sage.

Stevens, PJM, Schade, AL, Chalk, B & Slevin, ODA. 1992. *Understanding Research*. Edinburgh: Champion Press.

Stevens-Barnum, BJ. 1990. *Nursing Theory – Analysis, Application, Evaluation*. Glenview, Illinois: Scott, Foresman/Little Brown.

Strauss, A & Corbin, J. 1990. *Basics of Qualitative Research*. Newbury Park, California: Sage.

Streubert, HJ & Carpenter, R. 1999. *Qualitative Research in Nursing: Advancing the Humanistic Imperative*, 2 ed. Philadelphia: Lippincott.

Streubert Speziale, HJ & Carpenter, DR. 2005. *Qualitative Research in Nursing: Advancing the Humanistic Imperative*, 3 ed. Philadelphia: Lippincott.

Struwig, FW & Stead, GB. 2001. *Planning, Designing and Reporting Research*. Cape Town: Pearson Education.

Sweeney, MA & Olivieri, P. 1981. *An Introduction to Nursing Research*. Philadelphia: Lippincott.

Talbot, LA. 1995. *Principles and Practice of Nursing Research*. St Louis: Mosby.

Terre Blache, M & Durrheim, K. 1999. *Research in Practice: Applied Methods for the Social Sciences*. Cape Town: University of Cape Town Press.

Tesch, R. 1991. Computer programs that assist in the analysis of qualitative data: An overview. *Qualitative Health Research* 1(3), 309–25.

Thomas, BS. 1990. *Nursing Research: An Experiential Approach*. St Louis: Mosby.

Treece, EW & Treece, JW. 1986. *Elements of Research in Health Care Sciences*. St Louis: Mosby.

Trinder, L & Reynolds, S (eds.). 2001. *Evidence-based Practice: A Critical Appraisal*. Oxford: Blackwell Science.

Van Kaam, A. 1969. *Existential Foundations of Psychology*. New York: Doubleday.

Van Manen, M. 1990. *Researching Lived Experiences*. New York: State University of New York.

Van Zwanenberg, T & Harrison, J. 2000. *Clinical Governance in Primary Care*. Oxon: Radcliffe Medical Press.

Villaruil, AM. 1995. Mexican-American cultural meanings, expressions, self-care and dependent care actions associated with experiences of pain. *Research in Nursing and Health* 18(5), 427–36.

Walker, LO & Avant, KG. 1988. *Strategies for Theory Construction in Nursing*. Norwalk, Connecticut: Appleton-Century-Crofts.

Waltz, C, Strickland, O & Lenz, E. 1984. *Measurement in Nursing Research*. Philadelphia: Davis.

Wandelt, MA. 1970. *Guide for the Beginning Researcher*. New York: Appleton-Century-Crofts.

Wilson, H. 1989. *Research in Nursing*. Redwood City, California: Addison-Wesley.

Wilson, HS. 1992. *Research in Nursing*, 2 ed. Redwood City, California: Addison-Wesley.

Wilson, HS. 1993. *Introducing Research in Nursing*, 2 ed. Redwood City, California: Addison-Wesley.

Woods, NF & Catanzaro, M. 1988. *Nursing Research: Theory and Practice*. St Louis: Mosby.

World Medical Association. 1964. Human Experimentation Code of Ethics of the World Medical Association. Declaration of Helsinki: British Medical Journal (2), 177.

Yura, H & Torres, G. 1975. Today's Conceptual Framework within Baccalaureate Nursing Programs (Pub no 15–15558). New York: National League for Nursing.

Index

secondary sources 70
selection
    bias 98, 100, 126
    criteria, RCT 96
    of research problems 52, 57–65
selective retainment of data 40
self-determination, right to 31, 32
self-report
    questionnaires 142, 146–151
    techniques 146–155
Selye's stress theory 24
semantic scales 153
semi-structured interviews 152
sensitivity, instrument 165
settings, interviews 153
sharing data 31
significance of research idea 61
simple
    descriptive statistics 175–176
    hypothesis 83
    random sampling 127–129, 135
situation/-producing/-relating theory 21
Skinner's reinforcement theory 24
Solomon four-group design 95–96
snowball sampling 132, 134, 135
sorting 116
sources
    literature review 68, 71–74
    of research ideas 60
South African
    Medical Research Council (MRC) 31
    Nursing Association (SANA) 45
    Society for Nurse Researchers (SNR) 45
special technique sampling 132
specification matrix 148
split-half method 164
stability 118
    research instruments 164
standard deviation 178
standards for nursing research 45–48
statistics 68
    data analysis evaluation 186
    descriptive 171–182
    inferential 55, 171–172, 182–183
    parametric 182–183
    non-parametric 183
    sample 125
steps in research process 51–56
stratified random sampling 130–131
structured
    components, theory 25

interviews 151–152
observations 143–144
questions 148–149
study population 123
style, research report 193–194
subject factors, errors 159
subjects, research 51, 54
    availability of 63
summarising data 170
summated rating scales 153
summative evaluation 111
surveys 111–112
symbolic interactionism 10
systematic
    errors 158
    sampling 129–130, 135

table of random numbers 127, 128–129
taped information for consent 36
technical layout, research report 194
termination of research 47
testing
    theory 27
    threat to internal validity 100
test/refine theory 20
test-retest 164
themes, analysis 55
theoretical
    framework 19, 24
    perspective 19
    sampling 116, 132, 133–134, 135
theories, literature review 69
theory
    activity 18
    and research and research, relationship
        27–28
    critical 22
    definitions 19
    descriptive 19
    development of 25–27
    disengagement 18
    factor-isolating 19
    grand 19
    grounded 115–116
    levels of 19–21
    practice 19
    -related terms 21–24
    scientific 18–28
    source of research ideas 60
    testing of 27
    types of 19–21